The
Breast
Cancer
Handbook

The Breast Cancer Handbook

Taking Control
After You've Found a Lump

JOAN SWIRSKY & BARBARA BALABAN

HarperPerennial

A Division of HarperCollins*Publishers*

Breast Self-Exam art courtesy of the American Cancer Society.

Designed by Irving Perkins Associates

ISBN 0-06-095045-5

Dedicated to all the women who have traveled

the road from finding a lump to the diagnosis and treatment

of breast cancer and have inspired all who know them

through their fortitude, strength, and courage.

And especially

to Steve and Al

Contents

Introduction

by Joan Swirsky

In 1985 I was given an assignment to write a single article on the subject of breast cancer on Long Island. At that time, it had just come to light that this region, with its two counties—Nassau and Suffolk—had significantly higher breast cancer incidences than other counties in the state of New York. The state was about to begin a study to determine the "why" of this phenomenon.

From the first inquiries I made, it was clear that this mystery had many more questions than answers. That one article evolved into an eight-part series, during the writing of which what I learned both mystified and infuriated me. It was not long before I found myself becoming an "advocacy journalist," railing against a system that omitted important variables from its study, raising questions and suggestions that few wanted to answer.

But, as my monthly "Breast Cancer Updates" continued for months and then for years, some answers were forthcoming, the design of the state's study was changed (twice!), the environmental factors that were originally omitted were included, and I found myself invited to join advocacy groups and regional and state boards that were looking with increasing alarm at Long Island's problem.

Then, in 1991, I had a breast biopsy. With a sense of shock and dread, I realized that if I were, in fact, told that the biopsy was positive, I had no idea of what to do next! Armed with literally volumes of information and with my background as a registered nurse, I thought I'd be equipped to deal both intellectually and emotionally with whatever the outcome was to be. But that's not what happened!

What questions should I ask? What treatment should I choose? Should I opt for reconstruction? What if I needed radiation? Chemotherapy? Where would I turn?

The questions loomed large—the answers were nonexistent. I needed a road map, a "how to" manual that told me what to do. And, to my knowledge, none existed.

I turned to my friend Barbara Balaban and asked, "What do women do?" As if she had read my mind, she said, "Unfortunately there are no road maps!" In that instant, with that special unspoken language that like-minded people share, it was clear to both of us that we would try to fill this unmet need.

Introduction

by Barbara Balaban

The diagnosis (or even the suggestion) of breast cancer usually creates a state of crisis in a family. Amidst the confusion, the breast cancer patient has to learn a new language, understand her options and treatment choices, and make decisions quickly. At the same time, she must cope with fear, concern about her family, other people's attitudes, job responsibilities, and financial considerations. Because feelings of loss of control are among the most prevalent problems connected with dealing with breast cancer, it is important for every woman to take control over the decisions about how she will handle this disease.

As director of the Breast Cancer Hotline at Adelphi University's School of Social Work, I have seen how the volunteers who staff the hotline can restore a breast cancer patient's equilibrium and increase her ability to cope by taking her through the process step-by-step, with explanations and helpful hints.

It is my hope that this book will offer all women these empowering strategies, giving them information needed to make the best decisions possible about their breast cancer treatments; helpful hints that can make it easier to deal with the "little things" that can be so irritating; encouragement to take positive action on their own behalf; the belief that breast cancer is not a death sentence; some ideas on how to live a full, active life with breast cancer; and ways to take action to change the system.

Acknowledgments

We give heartfelt thanks to all of those generous people who encouraged and helped us with their referrals, comments, suggestions, advice, and support.

There are those whose assistance made this work possible: Stewart Kampel, editor of the *New York Times* Long Island section, referred us to Toni Mendez, our agent, who immediately saw the need for our book and enthusiastically and expertly guided us through the entire process. Peternelle van Arsdale, our editor, gave us the wise guidance the publication process requires. Very special thanks to Al Balaban, Cathy Bell, Diane Blum, Arlene Fell, Alan Garber, M.D., Sharon Green, Ellen R. Lande, Amy Langer, Ruth Liebross, Lee Naiman, Richard Shaffer, Eleanor Taub, and Vincent Vinciguerra, M.D., who read and reread the manuscript and made invaluable contributions.

Words cannot fully express our gratitude to Susan Love, M.D., for the generosity of her clear and erudite discussions with us about medical issues.

We want to make special note of the many other people without whose willingness to take action on behalf of breast cancer patients we would never be able to do the work we do: Jane Gitlin, publisher of *The Women's Record,* has published over a hundred articles by Joan Swirsky about breast cancer between 1985 and 1993; each and every one of Adelphi University's volunteers at the Breast Cancer Hotline who unstintingly give of themselves so that others may be helped; the hotline staff: Cathy Bell, Ann Carney,

Lyn Dobrin, Sandi Kafenbaum, Julie Rosow, and Carol Russo, whose dedication and support make it possible for the hotline to function; Dean Janice Wood Wetzel and Associate Dean Roger Levin of the Adelphi University School of Social Work for their interest, guidance, and support; Senator Michael J. Tully, Jr., and the New York State legislature, who passed some of this country's most progressive legislation about breast cancer, and all the New York legislators who really care.

A portion of the proceeds of this book will be donated to the Breast Cancer Hotline at Adelphi University School of Social Work, whose volunteers provide guidance, encouragement, and "how to" assistance to the thousands of women with breast cancer who call them each year.

The Breast Cancer Handbook—Taking Control After You've Found a Lump is not intended as medical advice, and a disclaimer is made for use of medical information or results thereof. The book is meant to educate and empower and not be substituted for appropriate medical care. The authors have made every effort to secure the most accurate and up-to-date information. However, in this very dynamic area, research, new treatment options, and medical opinion change rapidly every day. Therefore, it is possible that new findings may negate some of the information contained in this book. Major breast cancer centers use procedures that are not universally practiced. Some of the information or questions we have included may not be necessary if you are being seen at a breast cancer center, but it doesn't hurt to ask. *Whose lump is it anyway?*

Prologue

Nothing—absolutely nothing—prepares a woman to hear, to comprehend, to cope with these words: "There's a lump in your breast—we have to look further!"

Fear, even panic, take over. Your mind goes blank or you think of the worst scenario. Your reasoning flies out the window. Your heart thumps in your chest. And you feel alone, afraid, and completely in the dark.

Questions flood you: "What should I ask?" "Where should I go?" "When do I begin?" "How will I tell my husband or lover, my children, my parents, my employer, or my employees?" Your world has just been turned upside down. You feel out of control, perhaps the most frightening feeling of all.

Today, however, a diagnosis of breast cancer is not a death sentence. True, a "lump," to most people, means cancer. And cancer, to most people, means death. And death, to all people, means the end of everything they cherish, hope for, are doing, hope to do. But it is also true that millions of people are living longer than ever after a diagnosis of breast cancer and that, in many cases, their lives are full and active.

To start with, remember that 80 percent of breast lumps are benign.[1] To find out if you're in the 80 percent or 20 percent group, there are steps that must be taken. We're going to help you learn how you can control much of what will happen.

You *can* control your treatment and make sure you have the best possible outcome. Without exception, we have found that breast cancer patients who are informed, aware, and involved

---

1. Benign: not cancerous.

in their own treatment choices have felt stronger and more in control of what is happening to them.

Today you have a lot of choices. There are some new words to learn, some new ideas to think about. The choices create questions; the questions require responses and decisions. We hope this book will help you make those decisions.

We will answer your questions and help you navigate the road from diagnosis to treatment to recovery. We hope to empower you to take your illness into your own hands, to convert your depression into productive rage, to become knowledgeable about the many choices you will face, and to proceed full-speed ahead in the pursuit of recovery. We hope this will serve as a guide for men with breast cancer, as well.

Travel this road with us. From the minute your doctor tells you, "There's a lump in your breast—we have to look further!" this book can help you know what to do, who to call, what questions to ask—in general, how to proceed in this breast cancer world of uncertainty.

We do not mean to tell our readers which therapies are the "right" ones but rather to present the choices available, so each woman can make the decisions best suited to her. At the end of each chapter, there is room for you to make notes. We strongly encourage you to write *everything* down. In a time of turmoil, you can forget questions you wanted to ask, or the answers to questions already answered. Bring this book with you to the doctor's office. Use it as a guide. Technical or clinical words are explained in footnotes and in the Glossary. Also, chapters will include "Helpful Hints" and questions to ask—the "how to" of negotiating the medical and emotional maze. You will notice as you read this book that many statements and suggestions are repeated several times. We believe that repetition aids learning, particularly in times of crisis. The Resources section can be helpful at every stage and can assist you in finding booklets or reading materials on biopsies, clinical trials, etc.

Let's start at the beginning of the road: "There's a lump in your breast—we have to look further!"

Chapter 1

"Oh My God, Is It Breast Cancer?"

If you . . .

   . . . are told there's a suspicious shadow on your screening mammogram[1]

   . . . feel something different or strange in your breast or armpit

   . . . are asked by your husband or lover, "What's this?"

   . . . experience pain in or around your breast

   . . . observe puckering around a nipple, dimpling of the skin, or a nipple discharge

   . . . see a change in the color of the skin or nipple

   . . . suspect that something *may* be wrong

   . . . worry about what you've been told, felt, experienced, observed, or suspected . . .

Don't panic.
But don't delay!
Take three deep breaths[2] . . . and check it out.[3]

1. Screening mammogram: a routine breast X-ray.

2. Deep breaths: for maximum effect, take a slow, deep breath through your nose until you feel your lungs fill with air. Then let it out slowly through your mouth to the count of 15. Repeat three times.

3. Even if you are pregnant, these rules apply. Pregnancy does not protect against breast cancer.

Notes

Chapter 2

How to Check It Out

1) Make an appointment with your family doctor, gynecologist, or a breast surgeon.

2) Call a breast cancer hotline. You will be able to speak with someone who will offer you emotional support and practical advice. Many will have a special understanding because they have "been there."

Toll-free 1-800-877-8077 in New York State

Toll-free 1-800-221-2141 in other states

Toll-free 1-800-ACS-2345

3) If you haven't had a mammogram,[1] get one immediately. This will be a diagnostic X-ray, because you have a symptom. See chapter 4, "Mammography."[2]

4) If you don't know a doctor, contact your local teaching hospital[3] or medical society for a referral to a breast specialist. Or ask your family physician to recommend someone who is experienced in treating breast cancer. Since information about breast cancer is changing every day, it is important for you to see an "expert"—

1. Mammogram: a low-dose X-ray of the breast that can often detect tumors too small to be felt.

2. Mammography: the process of taking a mammogram.

3. Teaching hospital: a hospital affiliated with a medical school.

someone who is familiar with the latest research and treatment options.

5) There is no rush! Make an appointment with the doctor of your choice. Since a waiting period is usually hard to bear you can get another opinion while you wait.

Helpful Hints

1) If you don't know a breast specialist, ask your family doctor or gynecologist to recommend one.

2) No doctor is perfect. S/he can make mistakes—whether in treatment choice, the way s/he talks to you, or forgetting to call you. Your best protection is:

a. A second opinion.

b. Asking as many questions as you can.

c. A notebook,[4] pen, and tape recorder to record and remember everything day by day.

d. Someone to help you listen—and question. It's a good idea to bring a trusted friend along with you to the doctor; in this case, four ears are better than two!

4. Notebook: see appendix A, "How to Create a Notebook."

Notes

Chapter 3

Getting Answers

In dealing with breast cancer, it is very frustrating not to have answers to many of the questions about the disease.

Sometimes you don't get an answer because your medical team has neglected to give you some information. Sometimes it's because there *is* no answer to the question.

It is important, therefore, for every patient to try to be as "in charge" as possible of her breast cancer treatment.

Helpful Hints

1) Write down any questions you have, and keep asking them until you understand the answers—or that there truly are no answers.

2) The best people to ask are:

your doctor

a second-opinion doctor

the office or oncology nurse

a breast cancer hotline volunteer

the resources at the end of this book

Information from other sources may be well-meant but not necessarily up-to-date or relevant to *your* particular situation.

3) When you're told, "We'll have the results (of a test or procedure) next week," and then you don't hear—CALL. Ask when you can expect to hear, and then call at that time again—and again—and again if necessary.

4) Lab results are sent directly to your doctor, as are mammography reports. We believe patients are entitled to get their reports in addition to the reports being sent to their doctors. Ask the lab whether they'll do that—or ask your doctor's office to tell the lab it's okay to give you the reports. Some states are working to change the laws so that patients who desire them can get their reports directly.

5) Remember that science changes very quickly and some things included here may have changed. Check with your doctor and your hotline volunteer.

Notes

Chapter 4

Mammography

Mammography . . .

. . . can be an "inside look" at what's happening in your breast.

. . . is best done by a skilled technician and read by an experienced radiologist.[1] Both should be specialists in breast problems.

. . . is the best test by which women over age fifty can decrease breast cancer mortality by 30 percent.

. . . is the screening technique most widely recommended by experts for detecting *early* breast tumors. It will see 90 percent of tumors, but not every one, and not every one early.

. . . is safe—especially when the equipment is "dedicated" (i.e., made especially for mammography screening) and checked regularly by a certifying agency. And X-ray exposure on dedicated machines is extremely low.

. . . is nothing to be afraid of.

. . . is a first step. When you suspect you have a lump you should always get a second opinion, even if the mammogram doesn't show a mass.

. . . is covered by insurance when done as a diagnostic[2] procedure recommended by your doctor.

1. Radiologist: a medical doctor who specializes in the interpretation of X-rays for diagnosis and treatment.

2. Diagnostic: a test to determine the nature of a suspicious symptom.

. . . is sometimes uncomfortable. But how long does the whole procedure take? For both breasts—two minutes! *Two minutes that can save your life!*

. . . is done in either of two ways:

> standing (at a dedicated machine with two flat plates);
>
> or lying facedown (with breasts suspended through an opening in the table)

Mammography is not . . .

. . . anything to fear.

. . . harmful. The X-ray dosage you receive is about equal to what you would be exposed to while driving in your car for seven hours. It doesn't damage your tissues and the compression of your breasts during the exam doesn't harm them.

. . . the final answer. Although a mammogram can show a lump, it cannot tell if the lump is cystic or solid. If the radiologist wants to determine whether it is solid or ful' of fluid, an ultrasound[3] examination may be done in the office. This is a short, painless procedure. If the lump is found to be solid and the doctor wants to explore it further, s/he will recommend a biopsy.[4] (See chapter 7, "The Biopsy.")

. . . perfect. Sometimes a mammogram will be normal even though you have cancer. If you have a lump, always have it checked out further.

---

3. Ultrasound: Also called a sonogram, this is a painless test using high-frequency sound waves to see whether the lump is liquid or solid. Solid nodules need further evaluation.

4. Biopsy: a procedure in which tissue is taken from an area of the body for microscopic examination.

Helpful Hints

1) Ask your physician (or the breast cancer hotline volunteer) to help you find a radiological facility known to be experienced in doing mammograms.

2) When you call for an appointment, ask if the facility is accredited by the American College of Radiology (ACR). (See Resources for the ACR number.)

3) Ask when the equipment was last inspected by an outside certifying team. If it has been more than a year, look elsewhere.

4) Ask how many mammograms the facility does. If you live in a big city and the answer is less than ten per week, it may not be the most experienced place.

5) Ask if the radiologist will be there during your appointment. This is a diagnostic (not a screening) mammogram, and the radiologist should be present during your visit.

6) If cost is a problem, you can ask the doctor to accept what the insurance company pays.

7) For information about free or low-cost mammography, call your breast cancer hotline, the local medical society, the American Cancer Society, or a county hospital.

8) Before going for a mammogram, do not use deodorant or talcum powder because they may change the appearance of the X-ray picture. If you're offered an appointment immediately and have used any of these substances, tell the doctor.

9) If you feel the need for emotional support, ask someone to go with you.

10) Write down your relevant medical history, with dates, before you go so that you will be sure to tell the doctor all the important information. When you're in the office and feeling anxious you might forget some important details.

11) Find out if you have any family history of breast cancer, and at what age it was found. In previous generations this information was sometimes a well-kept secret, but the information can help in determining your risk.

12) Begin to record everything in your notebook! Dates, names, phone numbers, suggestions (and who made them), whatever might be important. This resource that you create will be invaluable to you!

13) Bring your medical insurance card or form with you.

14) Bring with you the name, address, and phone number of the physician to whom you want the official mammography report sent.

15) Although many places will tell you the results of your mammogram right away, not all will. The report will be sent to the physician you name (usually your family doctor, gynecologist, or breast surgeon). Ask *when* the report will be sent to your doctor.

16) If you've had a mammogram before, get the most recent films to take with you. If the radiologist only wants to give you a copy of your old films, tell him/her you are entitled to the originals (by law) and will contact a lawyer to obtain them if necessary.

17) Start to record your medical history. Include:

general health information

dates you noticed anything different in your breasts

tests done—when, where, and by whom

reports—written and verbal

and add to the list as you go along.

18) Don't expect a lot of understanding and sensitivity in this type of center. A mammography facility is sometimes more like a laboratory than a doctor's office.

19) If it will make you feel more comfortable, bring a friend.

20) Bring your notebook and pen to write down any information you receive.

Notes

Chapter 5

The Mammography Report: Getting a Diagnosis

There are two different reports: the doctor's *initial impression* (when s/he first looks at the films) and the written report that is completed after careful study of the films. Sometimes these reports are different. It is the second, more carefully studied report, that the radiologist will send to your doctor.

If the radiologist asks you to return for another set of films, don't panic! There are many technical reasons why this may be necessary. Whatever you have to face will be made easier by knowing the right questions to ask and by learning just how much *you* can be involved in your own treatment.

Helpful Hints

In all cases, we recommend that you get a second opinion!

1) Take a small tape recorder along because under stress you may not recall important information. No doctor should object to having his/her advice or information recorded—and you will be sure that you haven't missed anything. If the doctor does object, think about it—is this the kind of doctor you want?

2) If the doctor says s/he sees nothing wrong on the mammogram, but you still feel a lump, it may be because either:

the mammogram is not perfect, or

certain types of breast tissue tumors may not show up on a diagnostic mammogram.

3) A sonogram[1] is sometimes used as an additional check. However, the doctor may not always recommend further investigation. If *you* are anxious about still feeling a lump, insist on a sonogram. "Better safe than sorry" is a very appropriate attitude in this case. And of course, get a second opinion.

4) A lot of doctors try to aspirate the cyst in the office. If it's a cyst, it collapses and that's the end of it. If it doesn't collapse, further exploration is necessary.

5) Call your insurance company and ask if it will pay for a second opinion. Most insurance companies will. If you learn that your insurance company will *not* pay, you may need legal assistance. If you don't have insurance and cannot afford another doctor's visit, ask your hotline or your family doctor for help. (See chapter 30, "Dealing with Insurance Problems.")

6) Ask for a copy of the written reports. If your doctor won't give you a copy, make a handwritten copy from your chart.

7) Don't be afraid to ask the doctor to repeat something. For most people, medical terminology is a foreign language. It is common to have difficulty understanding

---

1. Sonogram: same as ultrasound.

everything you're being told, so ask again if you need clarification.

8) Select a special person to be your "care partner" or advocate. S/he should be willing to serve as the recipient of your fears and hopes, help with your own research, go with you to doctors, be your anchor. It should be someone who cares deeply but who can be objective and logical.

9) Call a breast cancer hotline. You can speak with someone who has been specially trained to talk with you, and may have had a similar experience.

10) If you have children and haven't discussed what's going on with them before this, do it now. There are books that can help (see your local or school librarian or suggestions in the Resources section at the end of this book).

11) Don't make the mistake of thinking children or grandchildren are too young to know. Children *know* when something's happening in the family. When you don't deal directly with your children their imagination goes to work, and what they imagine is usually worse than the truth.[2]

Go for another opinion—you're worth it!

---

2. See chapter 27, "Living Your Life as a Breast Cancer Survivor."

Notes

Chapter 6

Getting a Second Opinion

There is no *one* right choice of treatment. Each woman has to make the choice that's best for her at the time. The best choice is based on information.

Do it! Take your original X-rays, notes on your health history, and the first doctor's report to another physician. This can be a breast surgeon or radiologist.

If possible, select a doctor who is not associated with the same hospital as your first doctor. What you want is a fresh, objective view. A doctor who works at a teaching hospital may be connected to a medical school and may be more aware of new techniques and information.

Don't worry that the first doctor might be upset or angry that you want a second opinion. Most doctors welcome such consultations. If the two doctors agree—good. If they disagree, go to a third. Remember: it's in your best interest to be getting as much information as possible during this period. Also remember, a second opinion is no more likely to be "right" than the first.

If the films are "suspicious," you will need a biopsy[1] to know for sure what is happening in your breast.

Helpful Hints

1) Most insurance companies will cover a second opinion. Some require it. Check it out.

1. Biopsy: see chapter 7, "The Biopsy."

19

2) Take your notebook to every doctor's appointment.

3) Keep records of all your visits, including names, dates, the questions you asked, and the answers you received.

4) Remember to take all your reports and films home from the doctor's office. Save yourself the hassle of having to return for them!

5) It takes many years for breast cancer to develop. The "extra" time it takes—even several weeks—to get a second opinion won't make a significant difference in the outcome of your case, but it may make a significant difference in the doctor, hospital, and treatment you choose.

6) You can call the hospitals of your choice and ask for referrals to specialists connected with them.

7) While there is no formal listing of breast specialists, there are physicians whose practices are concerned mainly with breast care. (See chapter 12, "Choosing Your Surgeon.")

8) If you don't have insurance coverage, try to get a second opinion from another physician at a no-cost clinic or from another private doctor who works with a sliding-scale fee.

Notes

Chapter 7

The Biopsy

It would be an unusual person who would have a biopsy without feeling anxious. Your mind can race to the worst scenario you can imagine. You may recall all the stories you've heard and remember their worst aspects. Many women may think about their own mortality and imagine that their lives "will never be the same" if, indeed, a cancer is found.

Most women are so flooded with scary thoughts and overwhelming feelings that they don't know where to begin. "What should I know?" "What questions should I be asking?" "Where can I get the answers?" Before the biopsy you'll have many concerns, ranging from how the biopsy is done to whether it will leave a scar.

You may ask:

1) What is a biopsy?

A way to learn if tissues are cancerous or noncancerous. It involves the removal of the suspicious area for microscopic examination by a pathologist.[1]

2) How is it performed?

There are several choices.

> *Fine-needle aspiration:* This diagnostic procedure is done in the surgeon's or radiologist's office under local anesthesia. Several cells from the suspicious

1. Pathologist: a doctor who is a specialist in examining body tissue to evaluate the nature, cause, and development of disease. The doctor's written record of your biopsy findings is called the pathology report.

area can be suctioned out with a thin needle. If fluid appears and the lump disappears, that means it is a cyst and the problem has been taken care of. However, the mammography, pathology,[2] and clinical impression have to match, so if there's any question—for example, if the pathology report is negative but the lump is solid rather than fluid—the doctor will want to investigate further with a surgical biopsy (see definition below). Fine-needle aspiration is preferred if the tumor is thought to be benign, because it avoids surgical scars and decreases the number of incisions.

Stereotactic large-core needle biopsy: When there is a mass that can be felt or a lesion[3] able to be seen on a mammogram, a computerized X-ray pinpoints the lesion, and a wedge of tissue is removed from the area in question by a large needle. Since the sample of tissue is larger than that obtained from a fine-needle aspiration, many doctors believe its findings are more reliable. It is performed under local anesthesia by a radiologist or a surgeon.

Surgical (open) biopsy: The breast surgeon makes a small cut in the breast. If s/he removes only part of the tumor for examination, it is called an *incisional* biopsy. If the entire tumor is removed, it is called an *excisional* biopsy. This can be done in the doctor's office or in the hospital under either local or general anesthesia.

2. Pathology: the scientific study of disease, its causes, processes, development, and consequences.

3. Lesion: groups of cells or a mass; could apply to a lump, abscess, etc.

Note: The excisional biopsy is frequently preferred to an incisional one because it removes the entire tumor. Ask your doctor if you are having the excisional biopsy. If s/he says no, ask why not.

3)   Who does the biopsy?

We recommend that you go to a breast specialist who is familiar with this rapidly changing area of medicine. A radiologist performs the stereotactic biopsy and a surgeon performs the surgical biopsy. Your doctor should be experienced, have answers to your questions, know of the latest research in breast disease, and be able to discuss the many options open to you. If you can, get two opinions about your situation before selecting a doctor to do the biopsy.

4)   Does a biopsy hurt?

You may feel slight discomfort, but usually not real pain. It is a short procedure and, in most cases, you will be back to your normal routine within a day, or even several hours.

5)   Is tissue taken from just one spot or several?

Tissue is taken wherever there is a lesion.

6)   Are biopsies done on both breasts or just one?

Biopsies are done on both breasts only if there is an indication to do so.

7)   If a malignancy is found, will my breast be removed right away?

No, not unless it's necessary and you request it. If a malignancy is found, it is not necessary to perform surgery at the same time. Many women want to explore their options before deciding what treatment they will have. (See chapter 13, "Surgical Choices.")

8) What is meant by a two-step procedure?

The surgery is done in two steps: first, the biopsy; second, any further surgery that might be necessary will be done at another time after the biopsy. If the biopsy shows the presence of cancer, the two-step procedure gives you time to consider your options.

9) What questions should I ask the doctor about my biopsy?

What kind of biopsy am I having? Why?

What kinds of tests will be performed on the tissue?

How soon will I get the results?

10) Will I need any tests before I go for the biopsy?

If you are going to have general anesthesia, a series of routine pre-admission tests are required; usually they include a chest X-ray and blood test. You can get these tests anytime from a day to a week beforehand, depending on the hospital.

11) Do I have to be "knocked out"?

Usually not. The biopsy is generally performed under local anesthesia, sometimes along with a tranquilizer. The procedure takes fifteen to forty-five minutes. There might be slight discomfort. If the lesion is deep, you might get a general anesthesia that will either put you to sleep or sedate you, and will allow you to *not* remember anything about the procedure.

12) What is wire localization?

Wire localization is done before a biopsy is performed when the lesion can be seen on mammography but not felt. It is done with local anesthesia. Under X-ray, a tiny wire (about the size of a strand of hair) is placed in the breast at the suspicious spot to guide the surgeon in doing the biopsy.

13) Is the biopsy always performed in the hospital?

No. In some cases, the biopsy is performed in the doctor's office. Usually it is done in a hospital or surgical center, often on an outpatient basis, allowing you to go home the same day.

14) If I go to a surgical center or hospital, how long will I be there?

Several hours to a full day.

15) What is done with the biopsy specimen?

It is prepared for microscopic study. Sometimes the tissue specimen is flash frozen in liquid nitrogen so your doctor can receive a "first impression" report from the pathologist immediately. It takes longer to prepare the tissue for more detailed study. The final specimen may be available within twenty-four to thirty-six hours, although it occasionally takes longer than that for you to receive the findings. If the test is done on late Thursday or Friday you will probably have to wait until after the weekend before you obtain the results. Don't hesitate to ask your doctor to call the pathologist for the report if you are anxious about waiting (for up to a week) until your doctor receives it.

You might want a second opinion of the pathology. You are entitled to have the original slides for this purpose.

16) What about insurance coverage?

Biopsies are covered by insurance. Pre-admission tests are sometimes covered only if you are admitted as an inpatient.[4]

---

4. Many people have fought successfully against this. See chapter 30, "Dealing with Insurance Problems."

AFTER THE BIOPSY YOU HAVE A NEW SET OF CONCERNS:

17) How do I handle the seemingly interminable period of waiting?

There are several things you can do immediately. First, call the breast cancer hotlines:

Toll-free 1-800-877-8077 in New York State

Toll-free 1-800-221-2141 in other states

You will be able to speak with someone who will give you emotional support and practical advice—someone who has been exactly where you are now.

Then, try to do exactly what you ordinarily do in your social, family, or work life—don't miss a beat!

Right now, your goal is to *make the time pass.* Watch television, read, spend time with friends. You don't have to enjoy this time—all you have to do is get through it! This waiting period is probably the worst time—but you *can* get through it!

Also, start the habit of doing something special for yourself—*every day!* Take a walk on the beach, buy yourself a flower, indulge a fantasy.

If it helps you feel better to gather information about breast cancer, surgeons, oncologists, or various options for surgery at this time, do so. But if you think this is premature and you'd rather not discuss your situation with well-meaning friends, then remember—this is your right. Trust your instincts. Follow your feelings. *Whose lump is it anyway?*

18) Do I need a copy of the written pathology report and the surgical notes?

Yes. These reports are part of your medical records and you have a right to see them. It is important to have these reports available so you won't have to be subject to bureaucratic sluggishness to get them if you need them later.

19) When I receive the reports, what do they mean?

The pathology report is a description of the tissue. It will tell you whether the lump is benign or if you must take further steps. The surgical notes describe the procedures the surgeon used. These may be helpful if you have additional surgery (such as reconstruction) later on by a different surgeon.

20) What should I ask about the pathology report?

If it was benign:

What was it?

Was there any atypical hyperplasia?[5]

If it's cancer:

Is it cancer, precancerous, or in situ?

The size of the tumor.

How aggressive it looks (known as nuclear grade).

Whether cancer cells were found in the blood vessels.

Whether the cells were estrogen and progesterone positive or negative, and to what extent.

What the S phase is (how many cells are dividing at any-one time).

Whether cancer was found at the margins.

The answers to these questions are important because they will help you decide on treatment options.

5. Atypical hyperplasia: an overgrowth of cells that may increase your risk of subsequent cancer.

21) What do clear margins mean?

On the slides that are looked at, there are no cancer cells next to the edge of the sample. However, this is not definitive—there still could be some cancer cells that remain in the breast.

22) If surgery is recommended, what should I ask? Where can I get the information I need to make these decisions?

If your doctor says that the biopsy showed cancerous cells, that means you will need surgery to remove the lump and either part or all of your breast. (See chapter 13, "Surgical Choices.")

23) Should I get another opinion at this time?

Yes, if you have doubts about the report you've been given. Also, if there's a difference of opinion or if another hospital or doctor seems more desirable, you may opt for another opinion about the pathology. We *always* advise a second opinion before deciding on any treatment.

Helpful Hints

1) Ask the doctor beforehand what kind of anesthesia you will be having: a local, a local with tranquilizer, or a general.

2) Ask that the tests be done for estrogen or progesterone receptors. These can be helpful in indicating whether you might be a candidate for hormonal drug therapy later.

3) Request that as much tissue as possible be saved. Some hospitals do this automatically. It's your insurance that

enough samples will be available if you should need many repeated studies later.

4) Check with your doctor about the timing of your biopsy. There is some evidence that women who had breast cancer surgery performed between the seventh and twentieth day after the start of their last period were less likely to have the cancer reappear than women who had surgery before or after those days.[6]

5) On the day of the biopsy, wear comfortable clothing that's easy to put on and off, and low-heeled shoes. Even if you have a local anesthetic, you're bound to feel a little woozy after the procedure.

6) Don't wear any jewelry because you will be asked to remove everything except your wedding ring, which can be taped to your finger, if you wish.

7) Carry only a small pocketbook. All you will need are things like your insurance card, money for a taxi or parking, change for phone calls, eyeglasses, your house key, a small pad and pen, and some incidentals. Valuables are frequently lost during outpatient procedures.

8) You will be asked to remove your dentures and contact lenses if you are having general anesthesia.

9) Ask someone to accompany you. If you have the biopsy as an outpatient, arrange beforehand for someone (if not a friend or family member, then a taxi) to drive you home.

10) Bring your insurance forms and card with you.

11) Don't expect people to know what you want and need at this time. Tell them! They want to know! For

6. *Lancet*, October 1989.

instance, if you need help with transportation, dinner for the children, a substitute at work, or simply support and interest, let the appropriate people know. On the other hand, if you don't want to talk about the biopsy or how you're feeling, just say so. Most people understand.

12) If you have any questions, write them down, take them with you, and remember to ask them.

Notes

Chapter 8

"It's Benign! It's Over!"

Congratulations! Celebrate! Enjoy! You've just been through one of life's most traumatic events and you deserve to feel triumphant. However, don't be surprised if you also feel teary and upset. It's not uncommon for women to keep their feelings in check and then experience all the anxiety and depression after the fact.

Whatever your experience, go with it. Like the other milestones in your life, both good and bad, it will be something you are unlikely to forget.

Most women are not the same after having had a breast biopsy. It's usually a time to evaluate life, reevaluate priorities, and refocus.

Helpful Hints

Remember:

1) Have screening mammograms[1] regularly, on a schedule recommended by your doctor.

2) Have a physician examine your breasts every year, or more often if your doctor thinks it advisable.

1. Screening mammograms: see appendix C for screening mammography guidelines.

3) Keep your reports and notes in a special file. (There are many reasons why they may be helpful to a healthy person.)

4) Continue to be alert to any changes in your breasts. In spite of advanced technology in detecting tumors, most women find their own lumps. (See breast self-examination directions in appendix D.)

Notes

Chapter 9

"The Biopsy Is Positive—You Need Surgery"

Don't panic! There is no rush! Here again, the more you know, the better prepared you will be to cope with the days and weeks ahead.

At this point, you may find yourself flooded with questions:

1) How can this be? Last year my checkup was perfect!

Most breast cancers are there for eight or ten years before they are detected, but there is no way of predicting exactly when they will make themselves apparent.

2) Wasn't the cancer removed when the biopsy was done?

If the biopsy took out only a small sample of tissue now you need to remove the whole mass. And the doctor will probably want to remove some of the lymph nodes[1] under your arm for examination.

3) I don't understand. . . . I feel fine!

Great! Focus on that; it's a good sign.

4) What did I do to cause this? Why me?

One out of every eight women in the United States will get breast cancer in her lifetime. The causes are unknown, but we

---

1. Lymph nodes: glands under your arms that are usually examined to help determine the extent of the disease.

do know that many factors (e.g., genetic, environmental, etc.) are probably involved.[2]

Remember that you do not cause cancer. The causes of breast cancer are unknown.

5)   What do I do now?

Right now there are choices open to you and decisions to be made. Women find that as they begin to deal with the questions, the terror begins to subside.

There's a lot you can do. Stay with us.

Helpful Hints

1) There is no one "right" way. Each woman has to make the choice that's best for her at the time.

2) Keep in touch with your hotline volunteer. Now that you know your diagnosis, if there is someone who has had the same problem she can knowledgeably discuss the different treatment options you're considering, how you're feeling, and how you can begin to set priorities.

3) Take your time. While you shouldn't delay many months, you also shouldn't make decisions too hastily.

4) Get a second opinion. Take your slides and lab reports to a breast surgeon—preferably one at a different hospital than the one in which your own doctor works. Ask to have a second pathologist's opinion. (Reread chapter 6, "Getting a Second Opinion.")

2. Environmental factors: see Chapter 31, "Individual and Community Action."

5) Gather information about your disease. The more information you have and the more in control you feel, the better you will be able to cope and make the decisions that have to be made.

6) Consult the notes you've already made in your notebook, and if there are resources to contact, call them!

7) Call toll-free 1-800-4-CANCER to obtain medical articles and brochures about your condition and its treatments. It will be helpful if you know the stage[3] of your breast cancer.

8) Don't think badly of your doctor just because s/he's given you bad news. We sometimes tend to let that prejudice us against a good physician. Think about it—was s/he really abrupt in the way s/he told you? Or was there another way you would have preferred to get the information?

9) Your hotline volunteer can arrange for you to speak with women who have had the different kinds of treatments you're considering.

Note: When calling the hotline, ask for the same volunteer, when possible. She knows you and the details of your situation.

10) Think about installing call waiting, an answering machine, or a second phone. This way, when you're away or on the phone asking questions, you will be available to receive the calls that are being returned to you. A family discussion about scheduling telephone time can save everyone a lot of frustration.

---

3. Stage. In stage one, the cancer has not spread to the lymph nodes. Stage two is a small tumor that has spread to the lymph nodes. Stage three is a large tumor that has spread to the lymph nodes. In stage four, the cancer has spread to another part(s) of the body.

11) Don't be resigned to the notion that the cancer will defeat you. Breast cancer is *not* a death sentence. Be prepared to fight!

12) The best treatment choice is based on information. That's what we're going to help you find.

13) It's okay to be sad. But you also need to laugh. A sense of humor—even if it's "black humor"—will help. When a difficult situation arises, or you find yourself raging, try to find a way to laugh about some of the preposterous things you encounter. Read joke books. See a slapstick movie. Ask your friends to tell you their best—and their worst—jokes. There is good evidence from people like Norman Cousins[4] that laughter can have healing effects.

14) Physical activity engenders a sense of well-being. Find time to walk, swim, ride a bike.

15) Practice deep-breathing exercises or meditation as often as possible. These can be very relaxing and, according to some studies, can boost immune system function.

16) Guided imagery can be useful. While there is no clear-cut, scientific evidence of its benefits, many people believe it is helpful to develop a mental picture of how you are fighting your cancer, and winning! (See Resources under "Recommended Reading.")

17) If you have insurance, read your policy carefully. Make note of what time limits they give you for reporting, how to get forms, whether you need "permission" before going into a hospital.

18) If you don't have insurance, talk to your doctor or the office nurse about how to handle the costs of treatment. Ask about sliding-scale treatment centers.

4. Norman Cousins, *Anatomy of an Illness.* See Bibliography.

Notes

Chapter 10

Calcifications

With more women taking advantage of screening mammography, and because of new and better equipment, some extremely small lesions are being found. It can be very difficult to determine what some of these shadows mean.

If your doctor tells you, "There are some calcifications," you need to know more. Calcifications are small deposits of calcium; most are benign, some indicate the presence of a malignancy, and some are indeterminate. Some calcifications can be a marker for precancerous cells.

An enlargement of the films of the affected area (called a magnification view) can sometimes help define the nature of the calcifications. Benign calcifications are usually followed up by routine mammograms every year or two. Calcifications that are thought to be malignant require a biopsy (see chapter 7, "The Biopsy"). The calcifications that are said to be "indeterminate"—undefined—are usually checked again in six months. Precancerous cells are very slow-growing and a six-month delay probably won't matter. In any case, get a second opinion!

For calcifications that have not been clearly diagnosed, here are some of the questions you might ask to make your own decision:

1) Has a magnification view been ordered? If not, why not?

2) What are the chances that this type of calcification is malignant?

3) Is there a chance of scar tissue from a biopsy making it harder to see any future lesions?

4) What kind of biopsy will be done? Fine needle? Stereotactic? Surgical?

5) How will I handle the waiting period?

Helpful Hints

1) The kind of treatment you desire is your decision to make in partnership with your doctor.

2) Insist, nicely, on answers to all your questions. Trust your doctor to tell you the truth, but not to make your decision for you.

3) Second opinions, and more if necessary, are invaluable when calcifications are present.

4) Make sure the radiologist reading your mammogram is an expert with special training and a lot of experience reading mammograms.

5) Time spent considering your choices *now* can give you peace of mind *later*.

6) After a biopsy for calcifications, it is critical that you get a postbiopsy mammogram to document whether there are any calcifications left. This is necessary to assess any new calcifications that may show up on future mammograms.

Notes

Chapter 11

In Situ Carcinoma

In situ means "in place." By definition, this is precancer or noninvasive cancer that is contained.

What's so special about this condition? Because of the increasing use of screening mammograms, doctors are finding more of these precancerous lesions. There is a lot of disagreement among physicians about how to treat in situ carcinoma. That is why it is especially important to get a second opinion if your doctor says you have "in situ."

There are two types of in situ carcinoma; their names describe their locations. *Intraductal carcinoma in situ (DCIS)* is located in the milk ducts of the breast, the passages that deliver milk to the nipple. DCIS is believed to have a 30 to 40 percent lifetime chance of developing into infiltrating[1] breast cancer. Surgery (mastectomy or wide excision with radiation therapy[2]) is usually recommended, even though the lesion is very small and precancerous.

Lobular carcinoma in situ (LCIS), which is not even thought to be precancer but a marker, is located in the breast lobules, the deeper areas where milk production starts. It is believed to have a 20 percent risk of developing into infiltrating cancer over a lifetime. However, the cancer can develop in either breast; there is no way of predicting its course. Therefore, women with lobular carcinoma in situ are usually monitored carefully.

1. Infiltrating breast cancer: cancer that has grown outside of its original site into surrounding tissues.

2. Radiation therapy: the use of X-rays at high levels to destroy the ability of cancer cells to grow and divide. Both normal and diseased cells are affected. (See chapter 22, "Radiation Therapy.")

In the case of carcinoma in situ:

1) As always, second opinions are extremely important, since treatment depends on a proper diagnosis.

2) With lobular carcinoma in situ, mammograms should be scheduled yearly, unless your doctor recommends greater frequency.

3) With a diagnosis of intraductal cancer, you can take some time to investigate further before proceeding with any recommended surgery.

4) Adjuvant[3] chemotherapy is never indicated for carcinoma in situ, since it is precancerous and cannot have spread. Lymph nodes are usually not removed.

5) Hormonal therapy is now being used in clinical trials; its effectiveness is not yet known.

Helpful Hints

1) Ask the doctor which kind of in situ carcinoma you have. Different kinds behave differently and may determine the course of treatment.

2) Ask if you are a candidate for breast conservation surgery.

3) Ask what the margins are like.

4) Ask if the lymph nodes have been checked, and if not, why not.

5) Ask for a postbiopsy mammogram.

---

3. Adjuvant chemotherapy: anticancer drugs that are used in combination with surgery and/or radiation to prevent or delay the cancer from spreading.

Notes

Chapter 12

Choosing Your Surgeon

Choosing your doctor ranks with choosing your mate ... or your career. The choices you must make are critical—if not necessarily permanent—and will have a profound effect on your life. But you may be unsure you know all the things you need to consider in order to make the decision that's right for you.

Like the selection of your mate, you should have a strong, positive feeling about your doctor. However, unlike your mate, your doctor will not be as interested in making too many changes in his/her way of doing things to please you. Also unlike your mate, your doctor should want to be of service to you without expecting the relationship to be the proverbial two-way street. Most important, always remember that you are the employer and your doctor is the employee!

First, decide what qualities are important to *you*. Skill, of course. You want a doctor whose reputation in the field is highly regarded. But there's a lot more involved. Although you cannot personally evaluate surgical technique, you can evaluate the doctor's thinking about the surgery and the kind of approach s/he takes to you, as well as the surgical process.

You should always ask about doctors' credentials.

Are they board certified?[1]

What percentage of their practice is spent in breast care?

1. Board certified: they have passed a special exam in surgery.

Do they know about the latest treatments and studies that you may have heard about?

Here are some questions to ask yourself when deciding if a surgeon is right for you:

1) Does s/he relate to me in a way that makes me feel comfortable?

2) Does s/he talk to me in a way that helps me understand what's happening to me, both emotionally and physically?

3) Does s/he respect my desire to be involved in *all* the decisions about my care?

4) Does s/he use language I understand?

5) Does s/he have time for me—time and patience to answer *all* my questions?

6) Does s/he treat my questions seriously?

7) Is s/he open to discussing alternative treatments and other approaches (such as nutrition, vitamins, exercise) that might be of interest to me, whether or not s/he agrees with them?

8) Does s/he have telephone hours? When?

9) Does s/he, and the staff, treat me with respect and courtesy?

10) Are there any hidden questions, doubts, reservations, or feelings that I secretly have about the doctor that may hinder the kind of relationship I want?

11) What are my surgeon's credentials and has s/he been recommended by a doctor or friend whose opinion I respect?

12) With what hospitals is the doctor affiliated?

13) Is the selected hospital conveniently located for me?

14) Will the doctor and hospital accept my insurance?

15) Will the doctor adjust his or her fees if I can't afford them?

Helpful Hints

1) Trust yourself! Trust your feelings! Everyone wants the best for you and they've given you their best advice. But only *you* know what is best for you. Go with your instincts!

2) If you know a registered nurse who works in an operating room or on a medical/surgical unit, ask her or him for a reference. S/he will know how a doctor treats patients, conducts surgery, and regards women.

3) Ask as many people (friends and physicians) as possible for recommendations. See which names come up most frequently and which are recommended for particular qualities, such as compassion or experience.

4) For assistance in finding a physician, call your breast cancer hotline, the National Cancer Institute, the American Cancer Society, or your local medical society. A local women's health center might also be helpful. The nearest teaching hospital[2] or major medical center can provide you with a list of specialists.

2. Teaching hospital: teaching hospitals are affiliated with medical schools and are usually familiar with new techniques and information.

5) If you have reservations about your doctor, now is the time to consider a change. Think about it—and then, again, trust yourself!

6) Remember that no matter who you choose, nobody is perfect. Don't set yourself up for disappointment by idealizing your doctor. If s/he's not there for you at every moment, make sure that there are other available resources to answer your questions and support you.

7) Make a list of questions—your own and your family's—in your notebook. For instance:

What kind of surgery is recommended?

Why is the doctor recommending a particular choice?

Are there other choices?

Does my doctor do other kinds of procedures or just the one s/he is recommending?

What are the advantages and disadvantages of each choice?

How long will I be in the hospital?

Will I have any disability after the surgery?

Different procedures have varying success rates, depending on the type of cancer and how far along it is in its development. Since new research is constantly being done, and new statistics are being formulated on each type of procedure, ask your doctor:

Will my lymph nodes be removed?

What is his/her experience with my particular type of cancer?

What is his/her experience with each of the following treatments, both singly and in combination?:

Lumpectomy?[3]

Mastectomy?[4]

Radiation?[5]

Chemotherapy?[6]

Hormonal therapy?[7]

Nontraditional treatments?[8]

Note: Breast surgeons work with the oncologists who administer radiation, chemotherapy, etc., and therefore often have experience with them.

3. Lumpectomy: the removal of the lump and a small area of surrounding tissue. This is also called segmental mastectomy. It is often accompanied by axillary dissection.

4. Mastectomy (or modified radical mastectomy): this surgery removes all the breast tissue and some of the underarm lymph nodes. Muscle and nerves remain undamaged.

5. Radiation: localized X-ray therapy aimed specifically at the tumor and whole breast to cure or stop the spread of cancer.

6. Chemotherapy: the chemical treatment of cancer using drugs that kill cancer cells.

7. Hormonal therapy: chemicals given to block hormonal activity that may be affecting cancer growth.

8. Nontraditional treatments: all dietary (including herbal), meditative, spiritual, or religious and physical treatments that lie outside of those recommended by "traditional" doctors.

Notes

Chapter 13

Surgical Choices

Up to this point, you've made many choices. From the moment you felt a lump in your breast, or had a "suspicious" finding on your mammogram, you've managed to find your way in this new world—the new words, the confusion, the fear, the need to make decisions on a road you may have never known before.

Now, you wonder, "How can I decide what kind of surgery to have?" You're not alone in this decision. Your relationship with your doctor will be reassuring as you consider his or her advice and the experience s/he brings to your case.

Ultimately, of course, the choice is always yours. There is not one "best" choice for every person, except the one you, yourself, make. Your choice will be based on your lab reports, X-rays of various parts of your body, the medical advice you've received, the "homework" you've done, the people you've spoken with, and your feelings about what is *the best choice for you!*

What choices do you have?

- **Lumpectomy** (also known as *partial mastectomy* or *wide excision*). (See chapter 14, "Lumpectomy: Breast-Conserving Surgery.") Confined to a small area of the breast, this is surgery to remove the lesion and some of the normal tissue around it. It is the preferred treatment for early breast cancer. When a lumpectomy and node dissection are performed and followed by radiation therapy, the success rate may be better than that of a mastectomy.

- **Mastectomy.**

  Simple mastectomy. The surgeon removes as much of the breast as possible, but the lymph nodes and chest muscles remain.

  Modified radical mastectomy. The surgeon removes as much of the breast as possible and removes some of the underarm lymph nodes. Muscles and nerves remain undamaged.

  Radical mastectomy. Infrequently done anymore, this was the standard treatment for breast surgery for over fifty years. The skin, breast, chest muscles, and underarm lymph nodes are removed and most of the area is covered by a skin graft.

  Prophylactic mastectomy. A mastectomy performed to reduce the possibility of breast cancer. It may be recommended when a woman is at particularly high risk for breast cancer or for developing a tumor in the second breast after the first has been removed. If your doctor suggests a prophylactic mastectomy be sure to get a second or third opinion. When indicated, it is a reasonable choice, but not many women are candidates for this procedure. Counseling is always recommended for patients undergoing a prophylactic mastectomy.

- **Lymph node dissection.** During breast surgery, except in the case of in situ cancer, it is common practice to remove some of the lymph glands under the arms to see if cancer cells are present. The extent of lymph node involvement may affect decisions about later treatment.

- **Laser surgery.** The laser beam is another tool, used instead of the surgical knife. If you consider laser surgery as an option it is important to ask your doctor:

  Where were you trained in this technique?

  Can I speak to other patients who have had it?

  Why don't more doctors use this technique?

When it comes to selecting the type of surgery you'll be having, your doctor may feel that the location of the tumor and your personal history point to only one choice. Not all doctors may agree, however. In other situations, there may be several choices.

Remember it's your decision to make in consultation with the doctor of your choice—and no matter what, get a second opinion.

Each doctor has his/her own "pet" treatment recommendations, because the doctor's experience has found one to have a more favorable outcome than the other. Or, s/he may just be more comfortable with one or the other.

Some physicians believe that patients may do better with lumpectomy and lymph node dissection followed by radiation than with mastectomy. Some physicians, however, believe in the "take it all off" approach. The next two chapters will discuss lumpectomies and mastectomies.

ASK THE FOLLOWING QUESTIONS:

1) What type of surgery is the doctor recommending and why?

2) Why specifically does the doctor recommend the type of surgery I'm having? (You may know why *you* chose this option, but it's a good idea to review both your own reasoning and the doctor's before you proceed.)

3) What are the benefits of this type of surgery? What are the drawbacks?

4) What training has the doctor had and how many procedures like this has s/he performed?

5) What is the success rate of this type of surgery, according to the latest research?

6) What is the recovery period?

7) What side effects might I experience? What can be done about them?

8) What physical limitations will I experience immediately after surgery? Will they be short-term? Long-term? Temporary? Permanent?

9) Am I a candidate for breast reconstruction surgery?[1] If so, when would it be done and why? (Some women have reconstruction at the same time as their mastectomy; some have it later; and some elect never to have reconstruction.)

Helpful Hints

1) Now is the time to go through your notebook, look at all the recommendations and advice you've received, and check them out. Keep using the notebook to include new information.

2) Again and again and again, use the hotline! If you call once or a hundred times, there will always be someone there to listen to your concerns, share resources and

---

1. Breast reconstruction surgery: see chapter 16, "Preparing for Surgery," and chapter 19, "After a Mastectomy."

possibly first-person experiences, and give you additional advice, should you want it.

3) Review the information you've received from 1-800-4-CANCER. If you haven't called yet, call now.

4) Your family and friends want the best for you. But remember, their advice is only a suggestion—not a directive.

5) This is the time to get opinions from a medical or radiation oncologist about after-surgery treatments.

6) Once you've made your decision, trust it! And let go of any doubts.

7) Again, ask your doctor about the timing of your surgery. There is some evidence that women who have breast cancer surgery between the seventh and twentieth day after the last period have more of a chance of preventing recurrence.

8) Now, do something special for yourself!

In a few short weeks, you've . . .

. . . learned a new language.

. . . accessed resources.

. . . examined your own needs and desires.

. . . taken charge of what's happening to you.

. . . decided what's *best* for you!

You've done a terrific job!

Notes

Chapter 14

Lumpectomy: Breast-Conserving Surgery

For many women, the idea that they can have successful breast surgery without removing the entire breast comes as a great relief.

Other women remain uncomfortable about lumpectomy despite research—and the belief of many experts—that lumpectomy and lymph node dissection followed by radiation treatment is, for many women, equal to mastectomy.

Lumpectomy, followed by radiation, is sometimes known as "breast-conserving surgery," and is the treatment of choice for early breast cancer where there is only one tumor. This procedure, which is performed in the hospital under general anesthesia, removes the tumor and some lymph nodes, while leaving most of the breast. An area of normal tissue around the lump is also taken out to make sure that all the cancerous cells have been removed.

The procedure should only be performed by a surgeon experienced in the method, and a consultation with a radiation oncologist is suggested before deciding on the procedure.

Interestingly, at this writing, lumpectomies are performed more often on the East and West coasts of the United States than in the middle of the country.

For those women who are candidates for breast-conserving surgery, the advantages are many:

1) It is less invasive than mastectomy.

2) The postoperative recovery is easier, unless lymph node dissection is extensive.

3) The whole breast and most of the feeling in it are preserved.

4) There is minimal scarring.

5) The radiation treatments that follow lumpectomy are over in about five to eight weeks.

6) The side effects of properly administered radiation are usually not severe.

If you are interested in this procedure, question carefully any surgeon who tries to talk you out of it by saying that it's not as good as a mastectomy. Research indicates that when tumors qualify for lumpectomy, the long-term survival for women treated with lumpectomy and lymph node dissection followed by radiation is equal to those treated with mastectomy.

Some women ask:

1) Is lumpectomy a new treatment? Do we know enough about it?

Breast-conserving surgery followed by radiation has been studied for over twenty years, with consistent reports of its effectiveness.

2) How can I be sure a lumpectomy will "get it all"?

One of the problems with breast cancer is that we're never sure it's all gone, no matter what the treatment is.

Lumpectomy is used only in early-stage breast cancer, so that the chance of "getting it all" is very good. For insurance, a rim of healthy tissue surrounding the lump is also removed and, after the scar heals, the area is radiated to "burn out" any remaining problem cells. It is easier to radiate all the breast tissue than to cut it out.

After all breast surgery there is a chance that there may be a recurrence. Therefore, every breast cancer patient should be followed closely by her physician(s) so that any recurrence can be caught at a very early stage. When such recurrences do happen after a lumpectomy, the overall outlook has not been found to be any different than if you had initially had a mastectomy.

3) Will I need chemotherapy or hormonal therapy after a lumpectomy?

If, based on the information from the pathologist, there is reason to believe that the tumor has spread microscopically, chemotherapy and/or hormonal therapy will probably be suggested in addition to the radiation. If it is needed it can be prescribed before, during, or after radiation. Chemotherapy is sometimes given before surgery for certain early-stage larger lumps in order to shrink them to a size where they can be removed by lumpectomy.

You may wonder: Which is really better—lumpectomy or mastectomy? It depends on your body and your own wishes Consider:

1) What your doctor is recommending and why.

2) Which option offers you the best chance *today*.

3) Which decision you will feel more comfortable about having made three years down the line.

4) Which decision will allow you to sleep better at night.

After all, whose lump is it anyway?

Helpful Hints

1) Get as many consultations as you need to feel comfortable about your choice of surgery and your surgeon.

2) Ask your potential surgeon how many lumpectomies s/he's done for your kind of cancer.

3) Speak with a hotline volunteer about the pros and cons of lumpectomy versus mastectomy.

4) Ask to speak with someone who has had a lumpectomy, as well as with someone who has had a mastectomy.

5) Consider how much it means to you to retain your breast, or whether it's not important to you.

6) Whatever others say, it's *your* body and *your* choice.

Notes

63

Chapter 15

Mastectomy

Many women feel strongly that they want to "get it all out"—
that is, remove the entire affected breast. Unfortunately, even
mastectomy cannot remove all of the breast tissue, and nei-
ther a lumpectomy nor mastectomy can guarantee complete
success. Mastectomy is only indicated for multifocal breast
cancer, where the cancer is in several places in the breast, and
for women who have a large tumor (in either a large or small
breast) even if the cancer is in its early stage.

The modified radical mastectomy is usually done under
general anesthesia in the hospital. Halsted radical mastectomies are generally not performed anymore because removing the chest muscles is unnecessary and debilitating.

For those women who are candidates for mastectomy, it is
important to remember that:

1) It is the easiest way to remove multiple tumors in one
   breast.

2) Several choices are available for breast replacement.

3) If reconstruction is chosen, it can usually be done at
   the same time as the mastectomy.

4) Although it may be unrealistic, some women feel a psy-
   chological advantage in "having it all off."

5) Systemic therapy is often recommended after a mastectomy. This is known as adjuvant therapy. (See chapter 20, "Adjuvant Therapies," chapter 22, "Radiation
   Therapy," and chapter 23, "Chemotherapy.")

6) True lovers remain lovers.

7) There are hundreds of thousands of women in the country who are functioning well after a mastectomy.

8) Remember—you are a worthy human being with or without breasts.

As with all breast surgery, the procedure should only be performed by a surgeon experienced in the method. Some women choose to have a consultation with an oncologist before deciding on a particular procedure.

Again, one of the problems with breast cancer is that it's not possible to be sure that recurrence won't happen, no matter what the treatment is. All breast cancer patients are followed closely so that any recurrence can be caught at a very early stage. Recurrences in the mastectomy scar are often the first sign that further treatment is needed.

Helpful Hints

1) Get as many consultations as you need to feel comfortable about your choice of surgery and your surgeon.

2) Ask your potential surgeon how many mastectomies s/he has done for your kind of cancer.

3) Speak with a hotline volunteer who has had the procedure.

4) Remember, you don't need a breast in order to live.

Notes

Chapter 16

Preparing for Surgery

We hope by the time you're ready for surgery that you've spoken with your doctor about the various surgical options that exist and you're pretty well satisfied that you and s/he have chosen the best surgery for you.

There may be a feeling of relief at having made this important decision, but other questions—about the running of your normal life and about the hospitalization itself—remain.

Here are some questions you should ask your doctor about preparing for surgery.

1) Should I continue taking my normal medication (aspirin, vitamins, hormones, etc.)?

There may be a reason why you have to curtail or discontinue the use of certain medications prior to surgery. Aspirin, for example, slows down blood clotting.

2) Will I be able to eat before surgery?

When you receive general anesthesia, it is important that your stomach be empty to avoid the possible complication of throwing up undigested food.

3) When will I check into the hospital? Will I need any tests beforehand?

If your pre-operative tests are done ahead of time you will check into the hospital the day of, or the night before, your surgery. Tests may include blood work and a gynecological exam. Sometimes these can be done on an outpatient basis before your surgery.

4)   Who will give me anesthesia during surgery?

Either a doctor who is an anesthesiologist or a nurse anesthetist. Both require special training in administering anesthesia. Ask your doctor to arrange for you to meet the anesthesiologist before your surgery.

5)   What kind of anesthesia will I be having? Is it safe?

The anesthesia you get should be selected depending on the type of surgery you're having and your physical condition and makeup. If you are concerned, ask the anesthesiologist what side effects to expect when you awaken in the recovery room, and what risks there might be.

6)   Will I need a blood transfusion?

Not everyone does. If you have worries about needing a blood transfusion, make a real effort to donate your own blood—before surgery. In this way, should you need blood, you will be receiving your own safe blood. Don't ask relatives. They may not know their HIV status or, if they do, they may not tell you about their HIV risk.

7)   How long will I be in the hospital?

Some hospitals allow you to go home one day after surgery, or the same day, depending on the type of surgery. In some hospitals you will stay for three to six days. If you elect to have breast reconstruction, you may stay a few days longer.

8)   How soon after surgery will I see my surgeon?

Your surgeon should visit you within several hours of your surgery. In a university-affiliated or "teaching hospital," you will also be visited by interns and residents. If your surgeon has a partner, the partner may visit you if your surgeon is performing another operation.

9)   When will the bandages be removed?

This depends on your surgeon. It can take from twenty-four hours to a couple of days.

10)   Will I see a Reach to Recovery[1] volunteer?

If you are interested, discuss this with your doctor. Experiences vary depending on your locality.

11)   What kind of complications, if any, might I anticipate?

If you have general anesthesia the breathing tube inserted in your throat can make it sore. Sometimes drains are placed under the skin to help remove the fluid that has collected beneath the incision; this may last from three to four days up to a week. After a mastectomy there might be a collection of fluid under the scar. Occasionally, after a lumpectomy, there is a collection of blood in the tissues called a hematoma. One possible later complication from lymph node removal is lymphedema.[2] (For information about this condition, see chapter 24, "Lymphedema.") If you develop inflammation, tenderness, drainage, or fever, let your doctor know immediately. Depression and anxiety are also common. (See Helpful Hints at the end of this chapter.)

12)   When will I be able to resume my normal activities?

You may not feel like your "old self" for two to three

1. Reach to Recovery: a national program sponsored by the American Cancer Society in which women who have had breast surgery visit and counsel women after surgery, providing practical information, a temporary prosthesis, if needed, and some exercise suggestions.

2. Lymphedema: a swelling that results from the removal of the lymph nodes and the inability of the lymph system to drain fluid from the tissues. See chapter 24, "Lymphedema."

months after the surgery. You have had major surgery, which ordinarily is energy depleting.

In addition, you may have worries about the return of the cancer, finances, family care, etc., all of which can affect the period of recovery.

13) How soon will I learn my pathology results?

You should find out your pathology results in thirty-six to seventy-two hours.

14) What will the scar look like?

Breast surgery usually involves one incision; its location depends on the size of the breast. If you have had a lumpectomy your breast remains, but with relatively minor change, such as a slight indentation where the lump was removed. A second incision is made to remove the lymph nodes. A mastectomy scar is a line running across the area where the middle of the breast used to be. Over time, it will become increasingly lighter. If you have had a mastectomy, the surgery *does not* leave a hole. The skin that has covered your breast has been sewn together, so the area is flat, but smooth.

15) How long will it take for the incision to heal?

The incision for a lumpectomy usually heals within a week to ten days. For more extensive surgery, healing usually takes a month to six weeks.

16) How will I care for my incision?

Check with your doctor for specific instructions as to how s/he wants you to take care of your incision. Usually, within two to three days after the stitches are removed you can take a shower. If the stitches are not removed before you go home, the scar will probably be covered by a gauze pad for protection.

17) How soon will I know about future treatment?

If you have a lumpectomy, your doctor should have already discussed radiation treatments following surgery. The pathologist will look at the slides made during surgery. After your lab reports are all in, your doctor will discuss with you the number of radiation treatments s/he suggests and the possibility of other treatments, including chemotherapy. If you have had a mastectomy, you and your doctor will decide on further treatments after seeing the lab results.

18) Will I be deformed and uneven after a lumpectomy?

No. However, there may be an indentation in the breast where the tumor has been removed. The location of the tumor and the space where the tumor was will be quickly filled in by your body's own fluid, and the breast will retain its essentially normal shape and feeling.

19) If I have a mastectomy, will my appearance be unbalanced, uneven?

If you have large breasts you will initially feel unbalanced; small-breasted women generally feel less so. (See chapter 19, "After a Mastectomy.")

20) Can I have reconstruction after I've had a mastectomy?

The timing of reconstruction should be discussed with your doctor. It can be done at the same time as the mastectomy—or much later. (See chapter 19, "After a Mastectomy.")

21) Will insurance cover my hospital bills?

See chapter 30, "Dealing with Insurance Problems."

Helpful Hints

As you prepare for your surgery and try to learn as much as possible about the options you have, you will also be juggling

your personal and business life. Whew! Here are some suggestions that may help you get organized:

1) Hospital emergencies can cause the operating room to
be busy and delay your surgery—sometimes for many
hours. Ask your doctor to schedule your surgery for
first thing in the morning. It may be hard for you to get
there very early, but there will be less chance of a long
wait if the hospital gets busy.

2) Tell your family, friends, and co-workers what you're
going through and how they can help. Even if it's not
your style to talk about personal things, or ask for help,
this is a good time to change that. People care and want
to help! If possible, arrange for someone to carpool your
children, fill in for you at work, take over your errands,
etc. Then you can concentrate better on what you need
to do to take care of yourself. Also, let your children's
teachers know—they can be reassuring to the children
and better able to understand any unusual behavior.

3) If you're the boss at work, delegate temporary authority to a trusted colleague. If you're an employee,
speak with your employer about how much time you
will need to get back to your "old self."

4) If you don't get a lot of help at home, stock the kitchen
with easy-to-prepare meals. The more you take care of
things before your surgery, the less you will have to
think and worry about while you're recovering.

5) If you know your stay will be short, arrange for transportation home. You should *not* count on driving yourself.

6) Young children are reassured when the same person, if
possible, is filling in for you. If the "normal" routine,

including rules and discipline, is broken, children sometimes sense that something is seriously wrong. Try to prepare your child-care provider—whether your husband, babysitter, friend, or relative—in advance for how much of their time you will need, and how they can help to allay the children's fears. You can describe as much as you know about the hospitalization to your children, telling them that you will welcome their visits, and describing the things you'll be able to share together at that time: a card game, a book, television, and talking about the hospital and your cancer.

7) Call your insurance company before you go for surgery. *Many policies require you to tell them ahead of time.* Ask if you're covered for private duty nurses; if so, to what extent.

8) If your hospital stay will be just one to two days, travel light. A nightgown, robe, underwear, going-home outfit, cosmetics, toothbrush, phone numbers (yes! you can receive and make calls after the surgery—if that is *your* choice), and, of course, your notebook and pen. Try to bring front-buttoned gowns; they are easier to use with IVs or drains. Some women find a sweat suit comfortable.

9) When you look good, you feel better, so if you will be staying in the hospital for several days take along those articles of clothing and personal things that lift your mood and make you feel attractive. Pack a few pretty nightgowns, a bathrobe and slippers, a toothbrush, your cosmetics, and any other personal items such as photographs, magazines or books, an inexpensive watch. Also, if you wish, a deck of cards, a radio, a tape recorder

with a blank tape and earphones or a Walkman with some of your favorite tapes. But remember—security in most hospitals is a problem.

Note: If you've forgotten anything, a relative or friend can bring it to you, or the hospital might be able to supply it.

10) Don't wear nail polish. The color of your nails will be checked by the nurses and anesthesiologist as an indication of your general physical condition and circulation.

11) Bring a copy of your medical history with you, so you won't forget any important data. Also bring a list of *all* the medications you take.

12) Take your breast cancer hotline number with you.

13) Ask that a hormone receptor assay[3] be done on your tissue. This can be helpful in deciding on future treatments.

14) Find out what your blood type is. Write it on your medical history and also on a card in your wallet. Transfusions are usually not necessary, but should you need one, check that any transfusions match your blood type, and if you've banked your own blood remind your doctor and nurse about it.

15) If you sleep with a special pillow, or with a special noise-maker, bring these with you. Don't take contact lenses; regular eyeglasses are less likely to be lost.

3. Hormone receptor assay: a test to determine if your tissues are estrogen and/or progesterone positive or negative.

16) Although breast surgery is not considered a dangerous procedure, it's a good idea whenever you go into a hospital to write a health-care proxy or a living will,[4] leave some copies at home and bring some to give to your doctors and to the admitting office.

4. Health-care proxy or living will: a written form that describes how you want to be cared for if you can't voice your wishes and names someone to make treatment decisions for you.

Notes

Chapter 17

In the Hospital

Hospitalization is hardly an everyday event, so every question, every anxiety, every fear you have about it is normal. No matter how well prepared you are, you will probably still be wondering, "What should I expect?"

1) **Admitting/Consent Forms.** Your surgeon will give you "consent" forms to sign. You may also be asked to sign some general releases when you arrive at the hospital. If you read all the fine print—and you should—you're bound to feel anxiety. In essence, these forms ask you to agree to all the procedures and all the risks of the procedures that the surgery entails. *Make sure that the procedure you've decided on is the one listed on the consent form.* Also, be aware that unless it is stated on the consent form, another doctor may take the place of yours, should s/he have a personal emergency.

2) **Payment.** You will probably be asked to leave a deposit when you enter the hospital. *Make sure you bring your Medicaid, Medicare or insurance card with you.* You may be asked to leave a deposit in the amount of your deductible, or they may call your insurance company to find out how much of your deductible has already been satisfied.

If you don't have insurance be sure to find out ahead of time how much money you'll need to bring, and in what form (cash, check, credit card).

If you have any questions, ask them now! If you're having a lumpectomy, you will probably not be admitted as an inpatient to the hospital, unless you're having a lymph node dissection.

3) **Going for surgery.** After you've signed the forms, you will receive a plastic identification bracelet that will stay on your wrist until you are discharged from the hospital. Whether you are having a lumpectomy or mastectomy, you will probably go directly to a surgical or operating room waiting area and then to an operating room for surgery.

4) **Taking your history.** After you have changed into a hospital gown, the nurse, intern, or admitting doctor (or all three!) will take your medical and psychosocial history. This repetitious ritual takes place primarily in teaching hospitals. It is designed to reinforce already-known information and to learn new information that may be relevant—and it's part of a physician's training.

5) **Starting the IV.** Then the nurse or intern will start your IV, the intravenous[1] route through which medications and fluids are given. This is a short, mildly uncomfortable procedure that takes approximately ten to twenty-five seconds. If you count out loud, or pinch yourself, it will be over before you know it!

Note: Many patients, understandably, have anxiety about AIDS and wonder if it's dangerous to get an IV. The answer is no! All hospital personnel now practice uni-

1. Intravenous: the infusion of fluids directly into your vein.

versal precautions to protect themselves and their
patients when administering IVs or taking blood.

6) You will be asked to remove any dental bridges and
contact lenses at this time and to place them in con-
tainers that will be kept in the night table next to your
bed.

7) **Meeting the anesthesiologist.** Sometime before the
surgery, the anesthesiologist will visit you. Tell him/her
anything that concerns you. Be sure to mention any
medical condition you have, even if you believe it has
been noted already in your medical history.

Note: If you have *any* allergies—for instance, seafood,
dust, antibiotics, adhesive tape—or if you have an alcohol or drug problem, it is imperative that you tell the
anesthesiologist. It is important to be accurate about
your weight. Also, if you have anxiety, express it.
Don't think that anything is unimportant!

8) Your surgeon may visit you before surgery. This is the
time to tell your doctor anything that concerns you,
either physically or emotionally. Ask about medication
to help you sleep, and pain medication, if you need it.

9) You've already had your pre-op tests. Occasionally
some of the tests you've already had may be repeated,
such as blood tests. (You may also have blood tests after
surgery to check on your condition.)

Helpful Hints

1) Bring something with you to help pass the time while
waiting for your surgery. Delays are not uncommon.

2) Try to have someone with you to take care of your personal things.

3) Being in any hospital is a major assault on your emotions. Decide whether visitors and phone calls are what you want—and let people know.

4) If you have a health-care proxy or a living will, ask to have it added to your chart when you check in. Mention it to your anesthesiologist, your doctor, and the floor nurse.

5) If you think TV will help you pass the time, ask for it when you check into the hospital.

6) When you check in ask about having a phone connected, whether there is a special charge to turn it on, and what fees are for local, out of area, and long distance calls. Also until what time you are allowed to recieve and make calls from your room.

Notes

Chapter 18

Surgery and Postsurgery

You may either walk into the operating room (O.R.), or be wheeled in on a hospital bed.

Note: If you feel like it, you can chat with the attendant. Operating room attendants are highly experienced in their job and, whether male or female, they know what you're feeling and usually say those magical words that can put you at ease. Don't assume they are just a part of "the system." Sometimes their reassuring words make all the difference. If a family member or friend is with you, s/he may be able to go with you to the operating room doors.

The operating room itself looks like the kitchen you *wouldn't* want. It's a large, square room with tiled walls. In the middle of the room is the O.R. table and overhead is a big spotlight, the better for the surgeon to see what s/he's doing. In the rest of the room you will see cabinets (where supplies are kept), IV poles, and behind the table you will be lying on, the anesthesiologist's chair and equipment.

"I'm afraid of anesthesia!" Ironically, for some people facing surgery, this fear looms so large that it temporarily eclipses the fear of cancer. Actually, anesthesia "accidents" are rare. But this concern is why you've checked beforehand what anesthesia you will be receiving and who your anesthesiologist will be. And, until you receive the anesthesia, the operating room staff will tell you what they're doing and what you will be feeling to help ease any anxiety you may have. In addition, you will be closely monitored during anesthesia by an electrocardiogram, an oxygen pulse meter, and a breathing tube.

You will not remember the surgery. The anesthesiologist will administer a sedative through the IV that will make you unconscious during the surgery.

Then you will wake up in the recovery room. The most immediate sensation you may have is thirst. When the nurse gives you moistened gauze to suck on, it will taste great!

After a while, you will begin to feel discomfort in the area of the surgery—and the reminder that you've had breast surgery. Even then, the reality of the surgery may not sink in. You may still be too numb or groggy to understand what happened. Pain medications will help the discomfort.

After you've spent some time (usually two or three hours) in the recovery room, you will either be taken on a stretcher to your room, or be sent home. You may still be groggy, but after only a few hours you will probably be able to get out of bed to go to the bathroom.

Over your breast, you will see bandages that cover your scar and you will begin to realize that you no longer have the same breast that has been with you since adolescence.

If you stay in the hospital you might have an intravenous drip in your arm. Usually there is also a plastic tube that allows fluid to drain from the area of surgery. This drain may stay in for several days, until the area is dry and healing.

During your hospital stay, you will have doctors and nurses watching your postoperative progress. They'll be taking blood samples, checking your urinary output, blood pressure, pulse rate, etc. Every step of the way you have the right to ask them, "How am I doing? What do the tests say?"

If you look at your chart the following symbols might be of interest to you:

wbc = white blood count

hct = hematocrit (red blood count)

lft = liver function tests

BUN and Cr are kidney function tests: blood urea nitrogen and creatinine.

An "H" or "L" after a number means that the lab believes the counts to be high or low.

It's hard to give normal ranges for these tests because each laboratory has its own scale. For that reason you might be asked to have some tests repeated by your doctor although they've just been done.

If a Reach to Recovery volunteer visits you after your surgery she will know what you're experiencing. She's "been there"! She may be able to discuss your recovery with you—everything from simple exercises to prostheses[1] to long-range goals. You might want to call your hotline volunteer for some helpful hints.

If you're feeling pain don't hesitate to call the floor nurse. S/he usually has the authority to give you pain medication if you ask for it. (S/he may or may not suggest it unless you ask.) You don't have to wait until the nurse comes to your room on his/her own. In a busy hospital there is little time to spare, and the quiet patient is often ignored.

Friends and relatives, fellow workers, and neighbors may want to visit you while you're in the hospital. Some hospitals are strict about visiting hours; some are not. You might be happy to have a visitor stay on. But you may also feel tired or just not in the mood to be social, yet unable to say so because of the effort that person made to be there. Be honest! If you're tired, or not in the mood to see people, say so!

Whatever your feelings, respect them. This will be the first day of your healing process. You know better than anyone how you feel and how much physical and emotional energy you need to conserve. Trust your feelings!

And now, it's time for you to go home and begin to deal with whatever follow-up treatments your breast cancer may require.

Home is where "real life"—your family, children, job, finances, etc.—will face you, even as you grapple with the reality of your breast cancer, the possible follow-up treatments, the emotional highs and lows you may be experiencing, and the

---

1. Prostheses: artificial substitutes for any part of the body that is missing.

philosophical thinking in which you're sure to engage. (See chapter 27, "Living Your Life as a Breast Cancer Survivor"; also see chapter 20, "Adjuvant Therapies," chapter 22, "Radiation Therapy," and chapter 23, "Chemotherapy.")

After surgery, you may experience temporary (or sometimes permanent) numbness in the underarm area because during removal of the lymph nodes the nerves that control sensation in this area have been affected.

It is important to note that most women do not find breast surgery "painful." Uncomfortable, yes—but not painful.

Helpful Hints

1) Make an appointment for a follow-up visit with your doctor's office *before* you go to the hospital.

2) Any surgery is stressful to the system. Feeling tired after surgery is normal.

3) Before surgery, tape signs on your breasts: "On" and "Off." Although great care is taken to ensure your safety in the hospital, occasional mistakes are made. Women with whom we've spoken think that this "extra" precaution saves some anxiety.

4) Don't forget, *you* are your own best advocate. The more good questions you ask, the better your chances are of getting accurate and necessary information. If the doctors and nurses know you are an "informed consumer" they will be more aware of your need and your right to know.

5) Ask about the availability of a support group. This is an important source of emotional support and factual

information. Research has indicated that there can be physical as well as emotional benefits from participating in a postsurgical support group.

6) If you're going home with a prescription, make sure you get a supply of the medication you will need until you can get to a drugstore. If it's a holiday or Sunday, check to see which pharmacy in your area will be open, should you need to fill the prescription.

7) If you use your arm normally, without favoring it after surgery, you might be able to avoid any stiffness and you won't need any special exercises. Ask your doctor if you should be doing special exercises, and if so, when to start them.

8) Many women say they feel as though the breast they had removed "is still there." This is called "phantom sensation" and may last for a few weeks or for many years.

9) A copy of the surgery report from your doctor will be available in two to three weeks. Make sure you get a copy.

10) Ask your doctor about care of the wound and the surgical area and whether you should shower, use deodorant, and shave under your arm.

11) If you drive, ask your doctor if it's okay to continue right after surgery. You may not feel comfortable driving alone for a short while so, if possible, have someone accompany you or plan for other transportation.

Notes

Chapter 19

After a Mastectomy

A breast is relatively heavy. If you are large-breasted, you may feel it is important to replace the missing breast for cosmetic reasons, or to avoid a sense of imbalance. This can be done through temporary replacements worn externally *on* the skin (prostheses) or by more permanent replacements inserted surgically *under* the skin (reconstruction).

Some women want to achieve a presurgical appearance. Increasingly, on the other hand, there are women who don't mind the imbalance, particularly if they are small-breasted and not interested in wearing fitted clothing.

What you choose will depend on whether your particular body structure is better suited for one or the other, and your personal preference.

Reconstruction

Additional or lengthier surgery is required for reconstruction. Reconstruction does, however, give you the most "natural" appearance.

1) Who does breast reconstruction?

A plastic surgeon. Use the same care choosing a plastic surgeon for this procedure as you did your breast surgeon. Ask how many of these s/he has done. Membership in the American Society of Plastic and Reconstruction Surgeons is a good indication that the physician has received extensive training. And, again, get a second opinion!

2) When is breast reconstructive surgery performed?

Sometimes it is done at the same time as your breast surgery. It can also be done months—or years—after the surgery.

3) Does breast reconstructive surgery also include nipple replacement?

The nipple is restored in a separate operation, usually on an outpatient basis when the reconstruction is healed.

4) What options do you have if you are heavy-breasted?

If you're heavy-breasted, talk to your doctor about the possibility of a breast reduction on the other breast to keep an even balance. Sometimes insurance companies refuse to cover reconstruction. However, they may be required to by law. Call your hotline volunteer about the law in your state.

There are several kinds of reconstruction.

Implants

These are inserted under the muscle where your breast used to be. Sometimes an expander[1] is needed to make room for the artificial breast. Implants are breast-shaped bags filled with either silicone gel[2] or saline.[3] The outer covering is made from an artificial material, usually silicone. The long-term safety of a silicone envelope has not yet been determined. There are advantages and disadvantages to both kinds of implants. Saline

1. Expander: a hollow, empty sack that is placed behind the muscle and filled with saline over a period of months to stretch the skin before the implant is put in place.

2. Silicone gel: the liquid, synthetic plastic material used for implants.

3. Saline: a sterile salt and water solution.

implants may have to be replaced more often than silicone gel–filled. The silicone covering on implants has sometimes been known to rupture or leak. In the majority of women leaking silicone has not caused a problem, but some women are reported to have suffered serious autoimmune disorders[4] such as rheumatoid arthritis, lupus, or scleroderma. While there is no clinical proof about how dangerous silicone is and which women might be at risk for problems, the federal government has temporarily banned the use of silicone gel–filled implants (but not silicone-covered saline implants) for cosmetic breast augmentation. Breast cancer patients whose physicians recommend silicone implants can still get them if they join a clinical study that will monitor the implants' safety.

Sometimes scar tissue grows around an implant. This is not dangerous, but it can be uncomfortable. For some women the hardening is so severe the implants have had to be removed. Discuss the possibility of this with your doctor.

Signs of a ruptured silicone gel–filled implant include changes in the way your breast looks or feels, pain, numbness, burning, or tingling.

The most up-to-date information on silicone breast implants is available from the National Cancer Institute (NCI), the Food and Drug Administration (FDA), and the Breast Implant Information Network. (See Resources for telephone numbers.)

Flap Surgery or Surgical Reconstruction

Flap surgery uses tissue from your body to create a breast that is relatively the same size and shape as the breast that was removed. In a TRAM flap[5] the abdominal tissue is used and

4. Autoimmune disorder: a condition in which the body's natural defense system turns against the body itself.

5. TRAM-flap: transverse rectus abdominis myocutaneous—words that describe the anatomical parts of the body the surgery involves.

your abdominal muscles are weakened. Sometimes tissue from the buttocks (gluteal) or your back (latimus dorsi) is used instead. TRAM-flap surgery takes many hours and has a longer recovery period than implant surgery. While women enjoy the look and feel of this reconstruction, it does leave scars in the area where tissue was removed. As with any surgery, discuss the location of the scars with your doctor, and the pros and cons of this choice.

Prostheses

Removable prostheses make you look the same as you did before surgery when you're dressed. However, when undressing, the empty space and the scar can be a reminder of your condition. Also, the prosthesis has to be adjusted every day for comfort and appearance. It is important that prostheses be carefully selected and specially fitted to you. Specialty shops can provide this service; some communities have shop-at-home services available.

There are many different kinds of prostheses: heavy models held in place by special bras, lighter ones for sleeping or lounging. Paste-on styles have advantages but have been known to be less secure.

Your hotline volunteer can tell you about them. Usually prostheses cannot be fitted until a couple of weeks after the scar has healed. The Reach to Recovery volunteer can give you a temporary prosthesis.

Helpful Hints

1) Your hotline or the American Cancer Society may have free prostheses available.

2) Ask your insurance company whether they will pay for the cost of your prosthesis if the doctor has prescribed it. Medicare may pay 80 percent, plus the cost of some special bras.

3) There are several places to buy prostheses: surgical supply outlets, corset shops, some large department stores, and at-home services. Ask your hotline volunteer about the reputation of various prosthesis dealers. Be willing to travel to the best place rather than settling for a store that has a small selection.

4) There are several brands of prostheses. Find out how many different brands your store carries; the more brands, the more choices you have.

5) Ask whether an appointment is necessary, if there are private fitting rooms available, and whether and when a trained fitter will be in the shop.

6) Think about whether it will be easier for you to go by yourself, or if having a friend accompany you would be helpful.

7) At-home fitting services are more comfortable for some women, but the selection may be more limited and it may be hard to try a different brand if you're not satisfied.

8) Take your time. Selecting a prosthesis should not be rushed. Don't just "settle" to get it over with. Look in the phone book or ask your hotline volunteer for a corsetiere who specializes in prostheses.

9) Some prostheses come in dark and light skin tones so you can try to get one that best matches your skin.

10) Take a sweater and blouse with you to see how you will look in them. Clothing with horizontal stripes is helpful

in determining whether the prosthesis is sitting even with the other side.

11) Assess the attitude of the fitter. If you feel you are not being treated with the courtesy and attention you need, go elsewhere.

12) If there are special activities you want to engage in (swimming, running, dancing, etc.), discuss them—as well as your everyday needs—with the fitter.

13) If your doctor suggests that you wait a few weeks before being fitted for a prosthesis, look for "soft forms" that can be worn right away. Some forms are made with nipples; others can be worn with nipples that are sold separately.

14) There has been too much emphasis on "looking" at your scar. Look when you're ready, or if it's necessary. Some people find it helpful when looking at their scar to see positive images—a leafy vine, flowers, a pebbly path, a meadow stream, or even a humorous image.

15) Look, touch, and talk about the scar with your lover.

16) Ask your doctor or nurse to tell you how to examine your scar regularly. Report any rashes, lumps, enlarged lymph nodes, pain, coughing, or shortness of breath to your doctor immediately.

17) It is normal for some women to experience a "phantom breast"—perhaps an itch in a nipple or breast that isn't there anymore. This happens because the brain has not yet adjusted to signals from nerve pathways that, before they were cut in surgery, were accustomed to responding to certain sensations in the same ways over the years.

Notes

Chapter 20

Adjuvant Therapies

If your surgeon has suggested that you see a medical oncologist[1] (a cancer expert), it's to talk about systemic adjuvant therapy.[2] This is treatment after surgery when the doctors believe there is a chance that your breast cancer has spread or might spread. Choosing an oncologist is an important decision. You will have to deal with this person for many months now—and for many years in the future (although you are, of course, always free to change doctors).

Anticancer drugs, radiation or hormonal therapy are given either after breast cancer surgery (to prevent or delay recurrence of the disease), or before surgery (for the same reasons or to shrink the tumor in order to make surgery easier). The purpose of these treatments is to kill any stray cells that may have broken away from the breast and are growing in another part of your body.

You will want to know:

1) Should I have adjuvant therapy?

It's your decision. When it's recommended, most women do have it. The type of adjuvant therapy can vary with your special situation and with your particular doctor. Remember, get as many opinions as you need to make your decision.

1. Medical Oncologist: a physician specializing in treating cancer. There are medical, radiation, and surgical oncologists.

2. Adjuvant therapy: additional treatments after surgery, such as anticancer drugs and hormonal therapy, that help destroy any microscopic collections of cancer cells that may have traveled to other parts of the body.

2) If so, what kind?

Clinical trials. Clinical trials is the name given to investigational treatments that are being studied in controlled research programs at cancer centers and hospitals throughout the country. There are four phases[3] to clinical trials. Clinical trials give you the chance to see if new, not-yet-approved, treatments are useful to you. You also make a valuable contribution to research efforts by participating in the development of new treatments. (You may be among the first to get the next "wonder drug" or a new standard of therapy!)

If you're interested in being part of a clinical trial, discuss some of the following questions with your doctor:

- What are its advantages or disadvantages to me?

- Is the research approved by the National Cancer Institute?

- What phase of the trial is it?

- What side effects might I have?

- Will relief for side effects be available? To what extent?

- What are the results of this study to date?

- Will I have to go to a different hospital or doctor for this treatment?

- Will I have to pay for the treatment, doctors' visits, tests, or hospital care?

- Can I withdraw from the trial at any time if I choose?

<u>Radiation</u> (see chapter 22, "Radiation Therapy").

---

3. Phase I: trials to determine whether the treatment is suitable for humans. Before this all the trials have been done on laboratory animals.

Phase II: trials to determine whether the cancer actually responds to the treatment at all.

Phase III: trials that compare the new treatment with the best known standard treatment to determine which is more effective.

Phase IV: trials to adjust dosage, timing, and use with other treatments.

Chemotherapy (see chapter 23, "Chemotherapy").

Hormonal treatments. Because some breast cancer cells seem to thrive on estrogen, hormonal treatments are often recommended. They include:

Tamoxifen (Nolvadex®): a pill, taken twice a day, that prevents estrogen from helping cancer cells grow. Tamoxifen is the most widely used estrogen blocker today. Most women tolerate it quite well, but side effects of tamoxifen can include loss of appetite, nausea, hot flashes, depression, vaginal discharge, and headache. Some report short-term memory loss. Also, Tamoxifen sometimes increases the possibility of blood clots, uterine cancer, and possibly liver cancer. If you have a history of blood clots, tamoxifen might not be the treatment of choice. Women on tamoxifen should report any pains in the chest, arms, or legs to their doctor immediately, and should have a gynecologic examination at least once a year.

Megace: Hormonal medication used in the treatment of advanced breast cancer.

Surgery: sometimes suggested to remove the ovaries in order to stop the production of estrogen in the body.

DES: Used for postmenopausal women with metastatic breast cancer. (Daughters of women who took DES to prevent miscarriages a generation ago are at high risk for cancer of the sexual organs.)

Zoladex: Medication that stops estrogen production.

Autologous bone marrow transplants.[4] _This treatment is currently investigational for aggressive breast cancer._

---

4. Autologous bone marrow transplant: treatment using your own bone marrow, rather than marrow from a donor.

Chemotherapy agents are extremely toxic,[5] and particularly high doses can destroy healthy blood cells along with the cancer. To make treatment possible, bone marrow[6] is removed under anesthesia and stored for safekeeping while the chemotherapeutic drugs are given. It is then replaced when the treatments are over so it can make new, healthy cells. During this treatment the patient is vulnerable to infection, since the cells that fight infection have been removed. A growth factor (GMCSF) can assist in cell repair, shortening the hospital stay and reducing mortality.

Therefore, a bone marrow transplant requires a longer hospital stay than usual, under carefully protected conditions. Some hospitals allow children to visit.

With new technology it is possible to harvest some cells from the blood, rather than harvest bone marrow. However, it is difficult to gather many stem cells from blood and the technique may not be suitable for everyone.

Immunotherapy (also known as biological therapy). This method of treatment—*currently used only in clinical trials*—seeks to stimulate the patient's own immune system.

Other investigational drugs. Research is being conducted around the world because there is, as yet, no known cure for breast cancer. If you are interested in some of the latest research, discuss it with your oncologist,

5. Toxic: containing poisons (to destroy cancer cells).

6. Bone marrow: soft tissue in the center of bones where red and white blood cells are manufactured.

call toll-free 1-800-4-CANCER, and call or have your doctor call some of these researchers directly to see if their protocols are appropriate for you.

Note: The kind of research we are talking about here is being done by reputable physicians at well-known cancer research centers. These are not "alternative" treatments.

<u>*Alternative, nontraditional or holistic treatments.*</u> Increasingly, over the past decade, health-care consumers and doctors alike have begun to appreciate the "mind-body connection"—the degree to which thoughts, attitudes, and physical exercises, and therapies that alter them, contribute to a sense of well being and even improved health. If the idea of nontoxic treatments that are not generally accepted by the medical community appeals to you, take a look at them. These treatments have not been proven, but many have also not been disproved. Therefore, they are called *unproven,* or *nontraditional.* We believe these should only be considered in addition to, *not in place of,* traditional treatments, and should be discussed with your doctors.

For some people the idea of building the immune system through natural means is very appealing. However, if the publicity about the treatment sounds too good to be true, it probably is. Most of these treatments have not been tested in clinical trials or written up in reputable medical journals (where research is exposed to peer review and attempts at duplication). Vitamins and minerals can be helpful; they also can be harmful. Check them out with your doctor and with a nutritionist. Ask about side effects of large quantities. And ask why the traditional medical community hasn't accepted these ideas. Then make your own decision.

If you're interested in alternative, holistic, or non-traditional therapies, discuss some of the following questions with your doctor:

- **Has the treatment been based on controlled studies?**

- **Has it been reported in reputable scientific journals?**

- **Is it endorsed by qualified experts in the research community?**

- **Does it use blood? (This could expose you to HIV infection.)**

- **Can I speak to people who have had this treatment?**

- **What progress has the National Institutes of Health Office of Alternative Medicine made in evaluating this alternative remedy?**

- **Is it too good to be true? Remember—advertisements for these treatments are not subject to control. They can claim anything they wish without having to prove it.**

There is an important difference between non-traditional treatments that can be used with traditional treatments and those non-traditional treatments that are used as substitutes for traditional treatments.

Examples of treatments "used with" are guided imagery and nutrition; treatments that are relatively low profit, non-invasive and known to be helpful to many people.

Examples of treatments that are substitutes include coffee enemas and laetrile, which are often costly and frequently disputed.

When traditional treatments are found to be ineffective, they are dropped by government regulation. Non-traditional treatments are often offered "under the counter" or in a foreign country to avoid such regulation.

Alternative therapies may include:

Acupuncture. This ancient practice that originated in China involves the insertion of thin needles into special places in the body to relieve pain and treat illness. It can be effective for chronic pain, and has been gaining respect in some medical centers.

Nutrition. Special diets with vitamin and mineral supplements, aimed at improving the function of the immune system. (See chapter 21, "Nutrition.")

Herbal medicine. The patient is treated with herbs, flowers, leaves, and other parts of plants. (Note: many modern medications originally came from plants but are now manufactured from chemicals.)

Homeopathy. Extremely small amounts of highly diluted substances that are ordinarily used in higher doses are employed in this treatment.

Guided imagery. By using mental pictures, the patient is able to visualize images that help the healing process. This can be accomplished through (1) hypnosis or (2) relaxation training mental exercises that develop a sense of calm and ease tension.

Hypnotherapy. The induction of a trancelike state brought about by deep relaxation where the patient becomes receptive to suggestions that can be calming and relieve pain.

Biofeedback. The reduction of tension by becoming aware of involuntary body functions (such as heart rate, blood pressure, temperature, etc.) and learning to control them by conscious effort. It is effective for chronic pain.

If alternative therapies suit your beliefs and lifestyle, go with it! They can be healthy additions to traditional therapies. Not all of these are suitable for everyone, however, so check with your doctor about the possible side effects and how they will interact with your traditional treatments. Use them _with_, not as _substitutes to_, your treatment.

3)   Who administers adjuvant treatments?

A radiation oncologist gives radiation treatments. Medical oncologists deal with the various chemicals used to kill off cancer cells that may remain in your body after surgery. You will be working with your oncologist for a long time, so be sure you've chosen the one that's best for you. Check out as many as necessary. Consider the advantages and disadvantages of going to a popular cancer treatment specialist who may be far from your home, or to a well-recommended doctor closer to where you live or work.

4)   When will the treatment be reviewed to know whether it is working?

Different treatments take varying lengths of time before results can be measured.

Helpful Hints Before Treatment

1) Be sure to ask your doctor all your questions before making the decision to proceed with any treatment.

2) Your decisions about treatment should be based on what you think is best for *now*—not to hedge your bet against the "what ifs" of a later time.

3) Try to carry your notebook with you at all times. *Put your doctors' numbers on the first page, along with the number of your breast cancer hotline.* Use your notebook to keep track of how you are feeling and what medications you take and when. Keep a special section for the questions you think of between doctors' visits.

4) Depression and anxiety are normal after-effects of breast cancer surgery and treatment. This is a good time to find out if a cancer support group is available in your area. Some places have groups just for breast cancer patients; others for patients with various kinds of cancer. Call your hotline for information about a support group in your area.

5) See a nutritionist. There are many diets and supplementary nutrients that can help boost your immune system and keep your energy level as high as possible. Be sure to check with your doctor before using any.

6) Learn some relaxation techniques,[7] whether it's yoga, visualization, or just plain "tuning out" by picturing yourself at your favorite place of relaxation. It can relieve a lot of the tension.

7. There are cassette tapes for relaxation and guided imagery. See Bibliography.

7) Second opinions are very important before selecting a medical oncologist or radiation oncologist. Different doctors have different experiences and preferences in treatment, and there may be more than one acceptable approach to your particular condition. Also, you have to be content with your doctor's expertise, personality, hospital, availability for questions, and fee structure.

8) If you have insurance, ask your doctor whether your treatments are usually covered by insurance companies. Check with your insurance company about your coverage. (See chapter 30, "Dealing with Insurance Problems.")

9) People on radiation usually don't have to miss any time at work. Those on chemotherapy will most likely be able to do regular work between treatments, unless they are spaced very close together or you work at hard physical labor. Explain to your boss that you will be absent briefly, but will be able to carry out your assignment when you return. If you think it will be necessary to have your work load lightened, discuss that with your boss at this time. If necessary, ask your oncologist to speak to him or her, or send a letter. *It is illegal for you to be fired because of ill health.*

10) Find out what the "sick time" arrangements are at your place of work and if you can borrow against future sick time or vacation time should you need it.

11) Check with your oncologist about using your usual vitamins or medications. Some vitamins and medicine, such as aspirin and birth control pills, may not be advised while you're on adjuvant therapy because they may interfere with the effectiveness of your treatment.

12) See your dentist. It's a good idea to get all your dental work up-to-date before starting chemotherapy because side effects could interfere with dental procedures during treatment. Also, ask your dentist and your oncologist for some hints on mouth care during chemotherapy. Have your dentist call your oncologist for a consultation about possible oral problems. If you have a history of herpes simplex infections, ask about prophylactic treatment (Acyclovir is often used).

13) Ask your doctor about restrictions on food, alcohol, and activities, and what problems s/he wants you to report immediately.

Helpful Hints During Treatment

1) Make a list of the medications that will be prescribed and the dosage of each. Then check the name and dose before you take any medication, whether it's orally, by injection or intravenously.

2) Eating habits may be affected. While you want to maintain a well-balanced diet, it's more important that you eat foods you can tolerate.

3) Whenever you call your doctor's office, say what you're calling about and whether or not it's an emergency. If the doctor is not available, ask whether someone else can answer your question, or *when* you can expect a return phone call.

4) If you have a lot of questions to ask on your next doctor's visit, call the office and tell the nurse or receptionist that you will need extra time for them. If possible,

send the doctor your list ahead of time so that s/he can be better prepared to answer them. Bring a copy with you to the office so you can go over them together. If all your questions aren't covered during the visit, ask for another appointment to discuss them.

5) When going for your treatments, call the doctor's office before you leave home. Ask how the schedule is shaping up and whether you should come in as scheduled or a little later because of overcrowding.

6) Sleep is helpful. It can conserve and restore your strength. If you have a severe reaction to chemo, medication can help you sleep through it. Be sure to check with your doctor before using any medication.

Notes

Chapter 21

Nutrition

Good nutrition is always important, and researchers are increasingly studying the effect that different nutrients may have on the growth of cancer cells.

During times of stress, it is particularly important to eat well and provide your system with foods that will keep up your energy and boost your immune system. Many women have found that paying more attention to their diets has given them a sense of well-being and greater energy.

As always, we suggest that you discuss nutrition with your doctor, and ask for a referral to a nutritionist. These days, many oncologists work cooperatively with nutritionists.

Helpful Hints

1) Try to eat a low-fat but well-balanced diet. Fat is connected to estrogen production, and cancer cells feed on estrogen. In general, eating more plant foods and cutting back on animal foods will help. You can learn to read food labels in order to figure out how to estimate your fat intake. If you do eat meat, remove as much fat as you can.

There are many books and pamphlets on this subject (see Bibliography). A diet with less than 30 percent of calories from fat is acceptable; lower than that (20 percent) is good but may be too difficult for people to manage.

Some low-fat foods include: fruits, vegetables, whole grain products, beans, peas, and pasta. Look for the words "fat free," not "low fat," on processed foods. Avoid oil, butter, and whole milk dairy products.

2) Foods with vitamins A, C, and E are thought to be important. They are antioxidants, fighting harmful chemicals known as free radicals.

   Beta carotene is the plant form of vitamin A. It can be found in both fruits and vegetables that are usually yellow or orange in color. Fruits include apricots (fresh and dried), cantaloupe, honeydew, nectarines, mangoes, papaya, peaches, and prunes. Vegetables rich in vitamin A include carrots, sweet potatoes, corn, peppers, squash, soybeans, peas, black-eyed peas, and greens (turnip greens, romaine lettuce, endive, kale, spinach, and beet greens). Note: Don't overdose on fruits to the extent that you're taking in too much sugar. Too much of anything can be harmful.

   Vitamin C is believed to strengthen the immune system. It is also available in both fruits and vegetables. Fruits include the citrus fruits (oranges, grapefruits, lemons, tangerines), berries (strawberries, blackberries, raspberries, currants), guava, mangoes and kiwifruit. Vegetables include potatoes (with skin), tomatoes, green peppers, turnips, parsnips, asparagus, artichokes, and greens (okra, kale, collards, kohlrabi). Note: Overcooking can destroy vitamin C.

   Vitamin E helps keep cell walls healthy. It is found in vegetable oils, wheat germ, green leafy vegetables, eggs, and legumes (beans, peas, etc.)

3) Cruciferous vegetables in the cabbage family have gained a reputation among many researchers as cancer fighters. This group includes broccoli, red and green cabbage, cauliflower, and Brussels sprouts.

4) Don't let yourself get hungry. Fill up on foods with fiber. These include apples, bananas, berries, figs, dates, cherries, kiwifruit, papaya, and pears. Vegetables include beans, chickpeas, cowpeas, parsnips, plantains, and potatoes. Other high fiber foods are bran, multigrain bread, brown rice, and millet. Popcorn and pretzels have become favorite snacks—but be careful how much oil and salt they have.

5) Olive oil, canola and peanut oils are healthy sources of fat, in moderation of course.

6) Low-fat cakes are available in supermarkets and bakeries, and there are many fat-free frozen desserts as well.

7) Fish oils high in omega-3 fatty acids are thought to boost the immune system. Not every fish is low fat. Some fish that are known to have omega-3 include herring and sardines.

8) You don't have to give up all meat. White meat chicken, white meat turkey and veal are lowest in fat. When ground they can be substituted for meatballs or hamburger. For those who have to have beef, top and eye round cuts are leanest. Prime cuts have more fat than choice cuts of beef.

9) The use of vitamin supplements should be discussed with your physician and nutritionist. Overdosage with supplements can be harmful.

With all the other changes in your life, making changes in your diet can sometimes seem "too much." And eating—especially the "wrong" things—is often a great source of comfort during times of stress.

However, whatever you eat, try to make it well-balanced and nutritious.

Notes

Chapter 22

Radiation Therapy

Properly done, radiation has minimal side effects. The dosage and placement have to be precise for maximum effect without damage to surrounding organs. A radiation oncologist has been specially trained to work in this highly specialized field.

Lumpectomy is usually followed by radiation treatments. Mastectomy may also be followed by this treatment. Your radiation oncologist selects the dose and number of treatments you will receive, depending on the type, size, and location of your tumor. The treatments are designed to bombard the tumor and breast directly and destroy any remaining cancer cells. Most people function quite well during treatments.

Radiation therapy following lumpectomy is usually given five days a week for five to eight weeks. It begins about four weeks after surgery, after the wound has healed.

Each treatment takes only a few minutes, although there is check-in time and some waiting. Treatments are usually taken as an outpatient. You will probably feel well enough to get to the radiologist and back by yourself. There can be side effects during the treatment period, such as fatigue or a change in the color of the skin. Properly given, radiation should not damage nearby organs. Be sure to discuss possible side effects with your doctors.

Should you experience a cancer recurrence in the treated breast, mastectomy will probably be recommended. Reconstruction is an option, even after radiation therapy, although expanders may be a problem.

Radiation can also be given in conjunction with a mastectomy. Sometimes it is used to shrink a very large tumor to a more surgically manageable size, or to try to stop cancer cells from spreading before the tumor is removed. Radiation can be given after a mastectomy, either before or after chemotherapy to women who have had large tumors or many positive nodes.

Decisions about how and when to use radiation are made by the radiation oncologist. If both radiation and chemotherapy are suggested, you should ask your medical and radiation oncologists to meet together, with you, so that they can consult with each other about your treatment and how to answer your questions.

Radiation treatment is carefully designed for the shape and size of your breast. A few small identification markings (tattoos) will be drawn on your breast to mark the place where the radiation will be focused.

The side effects of radiation may include some fatigue, reddening and swelling of the breast, change in the color of the skin, and nipple soreness. Some breast tenderness might last for a long time—even years. Discoloration or tanning is usually temporary. Radiation sunburn can usually be treated with topical creams.

At the end of daily radiation treatments, internal or external radiation is sometimes given to the tumor site because that is the most likely place for a recurrence, if any, to occur. This is called a "boost."

Helpful Hints If You Are Having Radiation

1) Radiation might cause the same symptoms as sunburn: redness and swelling. A&D ointment may be soothing.

2) Be extremely careful not to expose a radiated area to the sun, especially for the first six months.

3) Avoid chlorinated pools or hot tubs during the period of radiation treatment.

4) Stay in touch with your hotline volunteer at this time. Many of them have discovered inventive ways of dealing with the aftermath of breast surgery.

Notes

Chapter 23

Chemotherapy

Chemotherapy is often suggested after a mastectomy or breast-conserving surgery, particularly if lymph nodes have been found to be affected or the tumor was large. This therapy—which can involve one, two, or even five drugs in combination—can be taken either by mouth, by injection, or intravenously. Treatments may last from four months to a year, or more. It can be administered in varying doses and at different time intervals. There are some protocols[1] that, after extensive testing, have become fairly standard for various kinds of breast cancer. Ask your doctor to describe your drugs before you start so you can be prepared to deal with them.

Yes, chemo can have some unpleasant side effects. Be aware that each treatment may have different side effects and that not everybody reacts to the treatments in the same way.

Some types of chemo are given in the doctor's office. Others are given in the hospital during an overnight stay, while some require a stay of several nights. Find out which arrangement is being suggested for you—and why. You will not only better understand what is happening but will be prepared to handle it and consider alternatives. If you will be staying overnight, ask about the kind of place in which you will be staying:

1) Can a "care partner"[2] be with you all the time, even overnight?

1. Protocols: a course of treatment using a specific therapy or combination of therapies.

2. Care partner: someone you choose who can be with you during your treatment.

2) Will you have to stay in bed or will you be able to walk around?

3) Can you wear your own clothes or are hospital gowns required?

Helpful Hints for Dealing with the Physical Effects of Chemotherapy

Note: Not everyone gets all of the following side effects.

1) If you experience a burning sensation during intravenous chemotherapy, call for help immediately. It may mean that the chemicals have leaked and the infusion needs to be restarted.

2) If you are pregnant, be aware that adjuvant therapy can damage a fetus. If you are not pregnant, it is important at this time to practice birth control. Chemo can cause loss of fertility in some women, so ask your doctor if your treatment can cause sterility. If so, some women decide to harvest and store their fertilized eggs for possible future use.

3) Premenopausal women may experience the menopausal symptoms of hot flashes and tenderness of the vaginal tissues. For the latter, use a water-based vaginal lubricant. Vaginal infections may occur. Use a non–oil-based lubricant and keep the area dry and free from chafing. Avoid nylon underwear or pants that are tight in the crotch.

4) Some women find their menstrual periods disrupted. Discuss with your doctor whether—depending on your

particular treatment and age—your periods will resume. (Do not assume that because your periods have stopped during chemotherapy, you are not capable of becoming pregnant during this time.) Women of menopausal age may enter menopause during or shortly after chemotherapy. Younger women may resume menstruation after chemo is over.

5) **Nausea.** There are medications that can help nausea. Ask how often these remedies will be given. If you will not receive them "as needed," ask why. (Some hospitals limit certain medications because of the expense.) Zofran is one of the newer, effective but costly anti-nausea drugs. It is now available in injectable as well as intravenous and pill form. Dexamethasone is not good for diabetics, but may help others. Compazine suppositories are very strong. If you know that you react to your chemotherapy with nausea or vomiting, ask for an anti-emetic to be prescribed *before* your chemo treatment. Discuss this with your doctor.

6) **Fatigue.** Fatigue is due to the temporary loss of red and white blood cells during chemotherapy. If the counts fall dangerously low, medications like Epogene may help, or a transfusion can help build them back up. Remember, if you are worried about a blood donor, you can donate your own blood before surgery.

Sometimes steroids (such as dexamethasone) are included with your chemotherapy to reduce side effects. This can provide a rush of energy that feels good, but can make it hard to sleep at night. After a few days, the burst of energy will be gone, and you may feel worn out until you rest and your body regains its normal energy level.

7) **Eating problems.**

Loss of appetite. Eat lightly before treatment; easily digested carbohydrates may be helpful. Ask your doctor for a food supplement if you're losing weight. Megace can increase your appetite. Milk shakes and crackers are often favored foods but avoid milkshakes if your stomach is unsettled. Avoid salted or fried food. Citrus fruits, roughage such as raw vegetables, and spicy foods can be irritating. Cool meats may be more appealing than hot ones. Arrange food attractively; eat with others; keep snacks handy; add nonfat dried milk powder to milk-based foods; drink juices and regular soda instead of diet soda.

Aftertaste. Avoid dry foods. You may avoid an unpleasant aftertaste by eating bland foods or rinsing several times a day with one part water mixed with six parts hydrogen peroxide (but not if you have mouth sores) or bicarbonate of soda. An unpleasant aftertaste can be reduced by sucking on hard candies, flavored ices, or ice cubes. Also, brush your teeth several times a day with a soft brush.

Food may taste differently than before while you're on chemotherapy. Eat often—five times a day—in small portions. Try plastic utensils because metal ones might affect your taste buds now. Test seasonings: they may not taste the same as before. Keep trying different things, but don't stock up on large supplies because your preferences may keep changing. You don't have to *enjoy* what you're eating, just find palatable foods that help you maintain your energy. Soups of various kinds can be nourishing and seasoned to suit your taste. Bland, hot cereals are often satisfying. Spreads on crackers can be tasty tidbits. A garlic taste in the mouth is a commonly reported side effect of autologous bone marrow transplantation. *Do not drink any alcohol unless you check first with your doctor.*

8) **Mouth sores.** Your dentist or oncologist will be able to tell you about rinsing your mouth and flossing to maintain dental hygiene during chemo. If you develop mouth sores there are several painkillers available—some lasting as little as twenty minutes, others several hours—that make it more possible to eat. Because you can bite the inside of your mouth if it is too anesthetized against pain for you to feel any sensation, be sure to check with your dentist and your oncologist before using any of these analgesics. Bland mouthwashes and cotton swabs can usually be used for mouth care. Avoid salt, peroxide, and mouth rinses that contain alcohol. An effective mouth rinse is 16 ounces of water, a half teaspoon of baking soda, and a quarter teaspoon of salt. Keep your lips moist with lip salves. Again, if you have a history of herpes simplex infections, ask about prophylactic treatment.

To coat your sore(s), pour some Maalox into a glass; let it stand and separate. Pour off the thin liquid and use the remainder as a paste. Rinsing with baking soda can be soothing. Avoid using stiff toothbrushes; rinsing and flossing are less harsh in a sore mouth.

When you have mouth sores, most people find that pureed foods, even baby foods, are easier to eat than whole food. Again, bland, hot cereals are often satisfying. Malteds, liquid food supplements, mashed potatoes, and applesauce are the kinds of foods that are easiest to swallow. Eat small portions, but try to eat so that you keep up your energy. Use natural vitamins and minerals as supplements.

9) **Mouth/throat dryness.** Carry sugarless mints or lozenges and a bottle of water around with you so you can take sips as needed. Also, ask your doctor about using artificial saliva. A substitute for artificial saliva is 8 ounces of water and five drops of glycerine.

10) It is important to control diarrhea with medication. Avoid fruits and gaseous vegetables.

11) Some foods, like cheese and rice, cause constipation. Ask your doctor about high-fiber foods, suppositories, and stool softeners.

12) Shortness of breath, weakness and fatigue, and blood in the urine or stool may be signs of a low red blood count and should be reported to your doctor immediately. Very black and foul smelling stool can indicate the presence of blood.

13) During chemotherapy, you may experience flu-like symptoms. If you have fever, chills, sweats, headaches, a sore throat, or severe coughing, tell your doctor.

14) People on chemotherapy are usually very sensitive to the sun. Protect yourself well—or better yet, avoid the sun during this period. Some makeup serves as skin protection for everyday use. Keep your lips moist with lip salves.

15) **Vein problems.** Because of the need for frequent IVs, your veins can become scarred or damaged. Ask your doctor about getting a mediport.[3] This avoids the necessity for repeated probing of veins. Use of this

3. Mediport: surgically implanted in the chest or arm, a temporary device to accept an IV. It may be accessed and used from one day to several days after placement, depending on the degree of healing (ask your surgeon about this), so it is important to think about having it done before serious vein problems start.

device is very much an individual choice. It does need to be kept clean and unclogged.

16) **Skin care.** Skin rashes may occur; your doctor can prescribe medication for these. To keep your skin from becoming dry and cracked, use lotions or oils. Wash your hands often. Chemotherapy after radiation can reactivate a radiation burn. Use cool compresses. Take warm baths (not hot) and dry yourself gently. Clean your rectum well but do not wipe vigorously.

17) **Hair loss.** Hair loss may occur with chemotherapy. It can affect all parts of the body, including arms, legs, underarms, the pubic area, as well as the head, eyebrows, and eyelashes.

Loss of hair is generally regarded as the most difficult adjustment you have to make. Some people find it easier to deal with hair loss if they cut their hair short prior to treatment. Others prefer to have a friend shave off all their hair at the start rather than dealing with the gradual loss.

If your doctor says that your treatment is likely to cause you to lose your hair, select a wig before you start chemo. (Get two if you can.) Also look at caps, turbans, and scarves as alternatives. If your doctor writes a prescription for a wig, some insurance companies will cover the cost.

There are various kinds of wigs: human hair wigs are the most natural looking; artificial hair wigs are made from synthetics, are less expensive, and need less care. Real hair wigs require the same care as your own hair. Artificial hair washes and dries more easily. If you get a wig, ask the shop about how to care for it. Wigs can come in standard sizes and colors or can be specially made for you. Select a color slightly lighter than your own hair; the thicker hair in a wig will appear darker than your natural hair.

Cost. When choosing a wig, consider the expense. Ask yourself, "How much can I spend?"

It may help to remember that your hair is falling out because the chemo is doing its job! Even if your hair isn't falling out, however, the chemo is working—not all chemotherapy causes hair loss.

Talk about how you look with your family, your friends, and certainly your hotline volunteer—and discuss "going natural" in front of them.

With some chemotherapy, a head "tourniquet" can be helpful to minimize hair loss; although it doesn't always work, it may be worth a try. Special ice packs may preserve hair follicles in some cases, but many oncologists believe that they also preserve other cells in the scalp, one of which might be malignant.

Some people find they get bad headaches from wearing wigs. Talk to your doctor about it, read up on it, and remember—it's your decision. Try turbans, scarves, or knit hats that you can color match to your clothes.

Definitely go to a "Look Good–Feel Better" seminar sponsored by the American Cancer Society and the cosmetics industry. Here, in a three-hour course, you will join other women undergoing cancer treatment and learn of new and helpful ways of applying makeup and using scarves to enhance your appearance. A call to your local American Cancer Society will tell you where these sessions are held—usually at your local hospital.

For hair loss (thinning), shampoo with a mild shampoo every two to four days. Use low heat when drying. Comb gently. Do not braid, get a permanent, or use hair dyes or rollers. A satin pillow (which is smoother than cotton) may help.

18) If your temperature rises to 101 degrees Fahrenheit or more, go for a blood count. If you don't have enough white blood cells to fight an infection, you may need intravenous antibiotics.

19) Call the doctor if you experience redness on your arms or chest, swelling of your arm, nasal or eye infections, or rectal or lip sores. These could be signs of important physical problems.

20) Your resistance is lowered during chemotherapy. Take precautions to avoid infection. Avoid cuts on your arms or fingers. Postpone your children's immunizations and stay away from children who have recently had inoculations. Wear a mask in crowded public places. Ask friends to tell you if they're not feeling well and, during those periods, to keep in touch with you by phone rather than in person. Avoid fresh fruits and vegetables, which can be full of bacteria. Don't pick your nose; blow gently.

21) Weight gain during chemotherapy is normal. This is not the time to try to control weight gain because you need a lot of nourishment.

Time for a Treat

1) Take time for a special dinner, a day in the country, an afternoon with an old friend.

2) Try to arrange coverage for your work or household chores and for transportation to and from therapy. You're starting on an important new road for you and your family.

3) A sense of humor will be important. You've made the best decisions you can. The difficulties that come up will be manageable. It won't be a totally smooth path, but you have the tools to make it work for you: hotline, second opinions, friends, and perhaps a newfound ability to indulge your own needs. Many of the problems that arise will be ridiculous. *Laugh!*

Notes

Chapter 24

Lymphedema

During or after breast cancer surgery some lymph vessels and nodes under the arm are usually removed. The job of the lymphatic system is to remove fluid from your tissues. Without the lymph nodes under your arm to do their work, the fluids may build up in the tissues in the arm. This can also occur if radiation has damaged the lymph system.

Not every woman who has a mastectomy or breast-conserving surgery develops lymphedema, but about 15 to 45 percent of women do. Lymphedema's symptoms can range from the mildly annoying to the severely uncomfortable, and require constant care. When your arm swells it causes discomfort and limits use. Infections can be difficult to treat, and dangerous. Because lymphedema changes your appearance, may limit your activities, and requires treatment, it can cause depression in some women. However, when properly cared for, it does not have to interfere with the quality of your life.

There is no cure for lymphedema, but the discomfort of the swelling, tightness, and heaviness can be managed effectively. Early treatment is always indicated. Lymphedema can occur anytime after treatment—even years later. This visible reminder of your breast cancer can be upsetting, particularly if it occurs later, after you thought you had the issue under control, or if it causes physical limitations. It can be helpful to remember, however, that while lymphedema requires vigilance, it is not a cancerous condition, and the procedure that caused the lymphedema also removed your cancer.

Some very specialized surgery is currently being tried and thought to be helpful for some women with lymphedema.

Helpful Hints

1) Soon after the surgery, unless your doctor tells you otherwise, try to use the arm where the lymph nodes were removed as normally as possible. If lymphedema is diagnosed, exercises are used as therapy.

2) Try not to stress the arm on the side of surgery where the lymph nodes were removed. Be a bit more careful about avoiding burns and insect bites.

3) Don't have your blood pressure taken in the arm where lymph nodes have been removed. (If you've had a bilateral procedure blood pressure can be taken safely under medical supervision.)

4) For both prevention and therapy, bicycling, walking, and swimming can be beneficial.

5) If swelling, pain, discomfort, or a rash develops in your arm, call your doctor for immediate treatment.

6) Do not try to treat lymphedema without consulting your doctor.

7) Ask your doctor about the different treatments to help lymphedema. (Some are not indicated for the patient who has an acute infection, congestive heart failure, or is on anticoagulant therapy.)

   Manual lymph drainage (MLD) is a special massage to remove lymph fluid from the affected arm.

   Compression pumps massage the fluid through the affected limbs and into undamaged lymph tissue. These can be rented or purchased.

   Air pumps perform the same function.

Special pressure "sleeves" and "cuffs" that control the buildup of fluid are often helpful. These sleeves force the fluid back into the lymph system and reduce the swelling.

8) Ask your doctor about the special elastic stockings that help keep swelling down.

9) Since infection can be dangerous, ask your doctor whether you should carry oral antibiotics with you, especially when traveling.

10) Although studies have never shown the following to make a significant difference, some people say they feel better following these guidelines:

Elevate your arm whenever possible.

Avoid extreme heat, such as saunas and hot tubs.

Take good care of your skin.

Maintain a low-sodium diet.

Wear protective clothing or gloves when you're doing something that may result in injury—gardening, using steel wool, handling hat pins, sewing.

Use an electric shaver rather than a razor.

Don't cut your cuticles.

Don't lift heavy objects or carry them over your shoulder.

Don't have injections, IVs, or blood drawn from the arm where lymph nodes have been removed.

Don't wear tight-fitting jewelry or cuffs.

Don't spend a lot of time in the sun.

Don't smoke.

11) If you are concerned about the appearance of your arm, loose, long-sleeved and attractive clothing—available for the summer as well as the winter—is recommended.

12) Some women find that air travel seems to worsen their lymphedema. Although the reasons are unknown, it is thought to be the result of immobility, the stress of travel, changes in cabin pressure, and the high salt content of airline food. If you are going to travel by air, the following suggestions may help:

   Bring your own food.

   Drink a lot of water and avoid alcoholic drinks.

   Stand up and move around during the flight if you can, at least every couple of hours.

   Wear a compression garment (such as sleeves or stockings).

   When making airline reservations ask for a seat where you can elevate your leg on a suitcase.

   If you tend to develop infections after flying, take your prescribed antibiotic twenty-four to forty-eight hours before your scheduled flight.

13) Exercise in moderation is important for lymphedema management. Water exercises in a pool reduce the stress on the affected area.

14) For additional information, write to The National Lymphedema Network, 2211 Post Street, Suite 404, San Francisco, CA 94115, or call toll-free 1-800-541-3259. They have a newsletter that helps keep you updated on the latest information about lymphedema.

Notes

Chapter 25

Hotlines

Breast cancer hotlines can be an invaluable source of information, support, guidance, and companionship before, during, and after breast cancer treatment. Many people are more comfortable talking about personal things over the telephone, rather than face-to-face. Phone calls are confidential and can be anonymous—it is not important to the hotline volunteer to know your real name; she just needs a name by which to recognize you if you call again, or if you should want her to call you.

One of the main advantages of hotlines is their availability. Some are staffed seven days a week; others just weekdays. But you don't need an appointment, and answering machines will record your message if the volunteer is away from the phone or busy with another call.

Hotlines don't charge for their service; the only cost is the price of a phone call and not even that if you use an 800 number. Hotlines usually have free brochures available to send you; ask for them.

There are two kinds of hotlines. The *basic support hotline* is useful for information, referral, and support. There is great reassurance in calling a hotline and learning that you are speaking to someone who has, herself, been through the same things you are going through. Most women appreciate being able to talk to someone who's "been there"--who has even had the same diagnosis, treatment, or side effects, and is familiar with all the things that are so new and strange to you. The most overpowering reaction that hotline volunteers hear is, "Wow! You've had breast cancer and you're still alive!"

Yes—still alive and working, running a household, being productive, and even having fun. The volunteers can be wonderful role models for you—reassurance that you, too, can get through this.

Most breast cancer hotlines are staffed by volunteers, many of whom have had breast cancer themselves. The best hotlines have required volunteers to take a course that trains them to find the resources callers need and to handle the various problems you may present from *your* point of view, not their own. These hotlines can usually help not only the breast cancer patient but members of her family as well. Some of these services have husbands, lovers, or children as part of their volunteer staff. Some hotlines are run by health providers and use professional staff to answer the calls.

Special *topic hotlines* offer help with questions on particular issues. For example, toll-free 1-800-4-CANCER is a government-funded service that provides information about cancer research and available treatment. The Lymphedema Hotline (see Resources) answers questions about this condition. These, and many others, are important sources of information in addition to your regular hotline. (See Resources for a listing of hotline numbers.)

Some of the breast cancer hotlines we've listed in the Resources directory have been in existence for as long as thirteen years. The reaction of women who have called them for help has been extremely positive.

Helpful Hints

1) Call a support hotline as early in your treatment as you can.

2) Call your hotline as often as you wish.

3) Give the volunteer a phone number where she can reach you in case she comes across some information you might find useful, or in case she wants to know if a referral she gave you worked out. Use any name you like.

4) Ask whether the hotline is run by a private physician or hospital. If a hotline is run by a hospital, as opposed to one that is completely independent (although perhaps housed in a hospital), it may not be as completely objective as one that's funded through grants and contributions.

5) While hotlines do accept donations—and are very glad to get them—they are not required and you should not be told to make a contribution.

6) If you are the kind of person who likes helping people and are good at it, think about joining a hotline yourself and sharing the knowledge you have gained through your own experience.

Notes

136

Chapter 26

Support Groups

In addition to getting the best possible medical care for yourself, one of the most important things you can do is join a breast cancer support group.

Getting cancer or losing a breast are life-changing events that involve a serious loss. Loss is life's most difficult challenge and the stages one goes through in accepting its reality are often painful and lengthy. A support group helps you deal with the loss.

Hundreds of thousands of women have found support groups to be life-savers in many ways:

- For the comfort of being with people who truly understand because they're experiencing similar challenges.

- To not feel alone.

- For the helpful hints you can pick up in handling your illness, the disease itself, and relating to family and friends outside the group.

- For the opportunity to talk about what's on your mind when you feel family and friends are reluctant to listen.

- Because research has indicated that breast cancer patients who are part of a support group might enjoy a better quality of life and live longer.

- For the ongoing network it provides when the support group is over. Special relationships are made in a support group, and they sometimes continue for years afterward.

- For the opportunity to know there's a place you can bring your questions and feelings each week rather than wondering how you're going to deal with them.

- To talk about things you're not ready to discuss with your family (for example, "What if my husband is telling me I'm still the same to him but deep down he's turned off?" or "I often think about my own mortality and don't know if I can discuss that with my family," etc.).

- For the chance to focus your worries and concerns in a definite time period each week. Some women find this gives them a place to go with those concerns that seem always to be in the back of their minds.

- To hear other women express feelings and concerns you thought only you had—and were afraid others might find foolish.

Even if you . . .
    . . . feel you have a good support system
    . . . are in counseling of some kind
    . . . aren't used to talking with strangers about personal
            matters
    . . . aren't usually comfortable talking in a group

Try it!

When you join a support group . . .
    . . . you don't have to join the conversation until you're
            ready.

... you don't have to talk about anything that's not comfortable for you.

... everyone is expected to honor each other's confidentiality.

Listening to what others have to say can be as helpful as the opportunity for you to talk.

There are several different kinds of support groups. Not all are available in every community. Groups can be either **time-limited**—usually six to twelve sessions—with everyone starting and ending together, or **ongoing**—in which people stay as long as they feel the need and new people join as others leave.

Time-limited groups are usually for people who have only recently been diagnosed or treated. Ongoing groups can either begin with "newcomers" or involve people who have already been in a time-limited group. In an ongoing group, discussion will generally be more like therapy groups, focused on the ongoing issues of dealing with the disease, with interpersonal relationships, and with how you feel about yourself and handle things.

Groups can be structured either as **topic-oriented** or for **open discussion.** In topic-oriented groups (which are usually time-limited), the leader has a schedule of which topics will be discussed at each session. In these groups you are sure that all those topics that are known to be of general concern will be covered. However, they often don't leave room for issues of special interest or immediate importance to be shared. Also, the leader of these groups has usually arranged to provide concrete information about each subject.

In "open" groups people can join at any time; in "closed" groups no one can join after the first one or two sessions.

Open discussion groups are freer, to allow members to bring up subjects of concern at any time. And members all learn from each other how to get their questions answered by the appropriate people.

Membership. Support groups can also be just for the patient herself or for **patients and family members together.** Close relatives can benefit as much as patients from groups; most are just as affected and concerned. It can also be helpful for patients and relatives to have a place where they can talk about issues related to the disease. There are other special kinds of groups that are sometimes available: couples' groups focus on how the couple, rather than the individual, is coping; groups for people who are experiencing recurrences; groups for the children of breast cancer patients; groups for spouses or lovers; groups for the very young breast cancer patient.

Group membership can be limited to just breast cancer patients, include people with all kinds of cancer, or be open to people with any chronic illness. Many of the problems that people with other cancers and other chronic illnesses have are very much the same as yours, so these can be very helpful if there are no groups in your area just for breast cancer.

Leaders. In some groups the group leader is a **professional** who has been trained in group leadership and psychotherapy. Other groups have **peer leaders**—usually people who have had breast cancer themselves and some informal training in group leadership.

Ask the following questions:

- What kind of group is this?

- Is it time-limited or ongoing?

- Is it open or closed?

- Is it topic-oriented or open discussion?

- How many people are in the group? (Twelve is the maximum recommended.)

- Is the leadership professional or peer?

- Are there just patients or relatives too?

Some women are concerned about support groups:·
"I don't want to hear other people's problems; I have
enough of my own." The act of helping someone else deal
with her problems increases your own sense of self-confi-
dence. Also, in hearing someone else working on an issue you
can apply some of the principles to your own life, even if the
actual facts are different. It's often easier to see what other
people are doing that's helpful or not than seeing the same
thing in yourself.

"I have a support group with my family and friends. I
don't want to replace that!" Family and friends certainly
can be your main support. But they, and you, will probably
also appreciate your having another place to go as well. With
their own concerns about you, family and friends cannot talk
as easily as other breast cancer patients can about all your
worries. And even if they've been through it themselves,
friends and family cannot be objective.

"If someone starts to cry I'm afraid I will too." We need
to cry, and crying with others is a special kind of sharing. In
our society we don't give enough importance to the value of
a good cry. There are plenty of times when you have to "keep
a stiff upper lip" (such as going for treatments and checkups); this needs to be balanced with time to "let it all out."

"What if the information I get is wrong?" With many people in a group the information is rarely *all* wrong. In any case,
you should *always* check information out with your doctor and
with your hotline volunteer.

Helpful Hints

1) Ask your surgeon, oncologist, the oncology nurse, or
   hotline volunteer to recommend a support group.

2) Support groups help you cope with your disease. They

do not take the place of psychotherapy, which helps people deal with relationships and life problems.

3) Talk to the group leader before you join to make sure that the group is the right one for you, and that you're appropriate for the group. If you have any concerns about joining the group (most people have at least some questions), ask the group leader about them before you join.

4) Most group leaders will suggest a trial period—an agreed-upon number of sessions in which you can try the group before making a definitive decision about whether or not to stay to the end.

5) There may be several different kinds of support groups in your community. Call around to make sure that the time the group meets, the kind of people in the group, the meeting place, and the kind of group you join best suit your needs.

6) If there is no support group in your area ask your physician, oncology nurse, or a social worker about starting one—or helping you form a peer support group.

7) If you don't have your own transportation, ask the group leader if one of the other members lives near you and can give you a lift. In some cases health insurance may pay for your transportation, or community agencies may be able to help.

8) Community agencies and hospitals usually have a sliding scale or no fee for support groups. Mental health agencies might charge a little more, but not as much as private practitioners.

9) While you will find people in your support group who have many of the same feelings as you do, not everyone

has exactly the same experience. Discuss any concerns about differences you have in your support group, and remember that you can get as much help from people with slightly different experiences as from people who share your experiences. They all know what fear, loss, and worry are like!

Notes

Chapter 27

Living Your Life as a Breast Cancer Survivor

"You're amazing!" As you find yourself getting back to life as you always knew it, perhaps going to work, raising your children, engaging in hobbies and interests, having relationships, and also going to doctors for checkups or follow-up treatments, this is a phrase you will hear often.

And you will probably shrug and say, "I'm not amazing. I just do what I have to do. What choice do I have?"

Well, you *are* amazing and, of course, you're right about doing what you have to do.

The trick is to do what you "have to do" in the way *you* want to do it. Considering the flood of advice you will receive from well-meaning people, it will sometimes be difficult for you to find your own voice. A good start is to continue the practice that you started when breast cancer was detected—making yourself informed, asking questions, getting answers, and trusting yourself.

You may find yourself still fearful, not feeling the relief you thought you would, but rather feeling like a cloud is hovering over your head. That's normal! Breast cancer is a challenge. Try to think of all the ways you've met previous challenges and summon them to help you now.

The first thing to do is to accept that your life will never really be the same. It can't be. There may always be that corner of doubt. "Symptoms" you once hardly noticed before—

headaches, backaches, arthritic pains, etc.—may now (and in the future) raise that awful question: "Has it come back?"

During this time, you may feel that a million things are pulling at you. The demands of children, household chores, going back to work, concern about finances, anxiety about whom to tell (and not tell) about your condition, fear of losing your job, and insurance reimbursement—all may make you throw up your hands and say, "This is too much." Well, maybe it is. This is the time to ask for the help you need. Chances are you've been "superwoman" for years, plowing through hard times and family crises and supporting others when things were "too much" for them. Don't do less for yourself.

In the Workplace. If your illness leaves you with any disability, the American Disabilities Act requires businesses to adjust the environment to meet some of your needs. You may worry that other employees may blame you for high insurance rates, but it may be helpful to remember that it's not your fault you got breast cancer— and the purpose of medical insurance is to cover you for medical problems.

Speak openly with your children about what's going on. Tell them if you're feeling teary or depressed. If you're sad or silent, they may worry that you're keeping something from them, rather than just experiencing a normal range of feelings.

Children's hidden fears are:

1) What did I do to cause my mother's illness?

2) Will she die?

3) Who will take care of me?

These are scary thoughts and often create feelings of guilt and anxiety in the child. Reassurance will help, even if these thoughts have not been expressed openly. Some helpful approaches for young children can include:

1) "We don't know what caused this. It happens to some people and scientists are trying to find out why."

2) "There are many ways to fight this disease and we are going to use all of them. Lots of people have this disease and live."

3) "You should be able to continue all your regular activities. For those days when I have to be away, who would you prefer to stay with you (or for you to stay with)?"

It's natural to ask teenagers to take on extra responsibilities at this time. That's okay; just try not to overdo it. Try to ask them which tasks they prefer to take on and let them be angry about it. After all, it does interfere with their freedom. And they're angry because this is happening to you, in much the same way you are angry. No matter how old they are, they probably have the same fears and questions as younger children do.

It's important to allow your children to express their feelings. Reassurance that you understand and that you're working on the problem is more helpful than trying to pretend there's nothing to worry about. They'll see through that—and will worry anyway. If you find it too difficult to talk, and even cry, about these things with your children, it might be worth finding a trained counselor to talk with them.

Speak with your children's school counselor, teacher, or principal. Let them know what's going on. It will help them understand if your child is cranky, upset, or "wool gathering." They can also keep you posted on how your children are managing away from home and alert you to any unusual problems. Some schools have special programs where children whose parents are ill can get together and share their feelings.

If you feel the need to talk, clarify your feelings, deal with your fears, or confront feelings of depression that may be hampering your energy (and your full recovery), then by all means seek help. Short-term therapy or counseling can be invaluable. Call your breast cancer hotline for a referral, talk to a psychotherapist, religious leader, or visiting nurse. Support groups can be extremely helpful.

And speaking of depression, that's normal too. It's almost impossible to go through serious surgery and any kind of follow-up treatment without struggling with feelings of depression, morbid thoughts, crying jags, and all the symptoms that accompany this state: loss of appetite, trouble sleeping, lack of energy, loss of motivation. Help is available. By all means, seek it out!

You may feel worse physically after your surgery and treatments than you did before. This is not necessarily because the cancer is worse; the treatments you've been through have been a rough road. You will need time to recover.

Breast cancer survivors say that the period right after their treatment has ended is a particularly difficult time. Before this, you've been busy taking care of yourself, searching for information, consulting with your doctor or team of doctors, dealing with work-related concerns and family and friends, juggling schedules. Now that the surgery and treatments are over and you are significantly less involved with doctors, hospitals, pharmacies, nutritionists, etc., you may experience an underlying fear and, strangely, a lack of relief. This may be the result of an unconscious anxiety: "Who's taking care of me now?"

The answer is that the team of doctors is still there. And the person who knows most about you is still in charge—*you!*

Measure your support system. If you don't think it's strong enough, ask your doctor, minister, local mental health agency, breast cancer hotline, YWCA/HA or school counselor how to improve it. They may know where you can find new social groups that will enlarge your support system.

You may still feel a nagging uneasiness because relationships with your husband or lover have changed. Some women say that just when you are feeling the most needy, the closest people in your lives—the ones you thought would be there for you—seem distant, or do not anticipate your needs or meet them. That, too, is normal. Most people find it difficult to face the issue of cancer; many feel at a loss about "doing the right thing." You may feel that the intimacy you shared, and now want, is not there for you. Again, try to talk about your feelings. And ask your partner exactly what feelings s/he has.

> *Note:* One good exercise is to sit across from each other and each express your feelings for a full five minutes, with no interruption. Each of you should repeat what the other has said before making his or her statements. In this way, you will both learn what the other one is feeling—and it may help to restore the intimacy that is missing.

You will probably be seeing your oncologist, breast surgeon, and radiation therapist regularly. Most women find their postsurgery checkups very traumatic, even years later. Returning to the hospital—or doctor—can cause nausea or severe anxiety. It's hard to think of this checkup as ordinary; after all, it's a visit to see if the cancer has returned.

Since this is your worst fear, it's natural to be nervous. Talk about it with a family member, friend, or with your hotline volunteer. Arrange the day so it's most comfortable for you. Ask a friend to go with you. Or plan a special treat for after the visit.

Survivors report that their lives have been totally changed . . . and often for the better! You may have a new perspective on things. Priorities have probably changed. For many women, this is a deeply philosophical time, a time for grappling with thoughts of mortality. It may be the first time you've thought about making out a will or revising an existing one. Again, these thoughts, rather than demoralizing you, may lead to renewed vigor for those things that are really important. Spending the time to speak with a friend or watch a favorite show may now be more important than doing a household chore. You may want flowers for your home or work place to fill that dark corner you formerly tolerated. A self-enhancing treat like a new scarf or a lipstick may be more important than a more practical purchase.

Keep a diary. A notebook of how you're feeling, both emotionally and physically, will provide you with a good record—one you may look back on with amazement and one that is useful for follow-up doctor's visits. It's also a great way to be able to express your feelings—the ups and downs—instead of bottling them up.

"So what?" you may say. "I know I'll be feeling bad—why put it down?" Because, much to your surprise, there will be many times that you don't feel bad; times you'll laugh, times you'll participate in events with good feelings, times you'll feel in control and good about it. And when you're feeling upset, writing it down is one way of getting it out—from the inside to the outside.

Sometimes, at a particularly low period, it is good to refer to the better times and even the reason why you felt that way. Often this allows you to see how your mind worked at a particular time, and to recapture that thinking in the present.

This is also a good time to make a list of your long-range and short-range goals. Share your goals with family or friends so they'll understand your decisions. Urge them to do the same. Generally, more time with special people in your life is high on the list. Take a special trip. Learn a new skill. Whatever it is, go for it!

Don't just let it happen—plan it. And to those well-meaning friends who have their own ideas of what you *should* be doing, learn to say, "Don't 'should' on me!"

As time goes by, you may find people don't want to hear about your lingering worries. "Put it all behind you," they may say. This is a good time to keep in touch with your hotline volunteer or support group members. They know it's never all behind you and they know how to listen.

Explain to your family and friends that when you talk about your concerns, you don't expect them to *do* anything about it—you just need to have them listen. If they can't, ask them what you can and cannot expect from them. Remember, people need to learn how they can be helpful to you. Don't assume they already know. You know how your body feels— they can only wonder and worry about you.

Helpful Hints

1) When you're worried that something new may be wrong, see your doctor. Listen to your body!

2) You may feel better if you stagger your follow-up appointments so that you're seeing each of your physicians every few months instead of all of them at once.

3) If the doctor wants to check your lungs, liver, or bones, s/he may do a CAT scan.[1] If you are allergic to the regular dye, ask for a non-ionic dye.

4) CEA and CA15-3 are two blood tests that are sometimes thought to alert your physician to early warning signs of recurring cancer. These tests are of limited use. There is no evidence that finding a recurrence early makes any difference in your treatment or your survival. You will be followed closely after treatments, and should you experience a recurrence, other treatments can put you in remission.

5) Expect fatigue and build in time for it.

6) Some women want to maintain contact with the latest information on breast cancer treatment, and some don't. Think about which you are and do whatever makes you most comfortable.

1. CAT scan: computerized axial tomography visualizes a specific area in cross-sections that can be examined separately. It can be done with contrast or without contrast—the latter gives a clearer picture.

7) If you think you need counseling, ask a trusted friend, your doctor, or hotline volunteer for a referral. It's best to see someone who is personally recommended and who has worked with breast cancer patients.

8) Nurture hope. If you experience a physical setback, remember that it may only be temporary. Most unpleasant side effects do pass. Each phase of treatment increases your chances for a good recovery. The new treatment that's just around the corner might be the perfect one for you. Find something to look forward to—promise yourself a treat of some kind.

9) Take things one day at a time. You've earned each one!

Notes

153

Chapter 28

Sexuality

If You're in a Relationship

Most women worry about how breast cancer will affect their sexuality and how breast cancer treatment will affect their sex lives.

You may feel a lack of sexual interest during and after your treatment. This is because your energies and thoughts are primarily directed toward your health. Fatigue is a major contributing cause, and many of the breast cancer treatments cause tissue dryness and loss of sexual drive.

At the same time you may feel the need for cuddling and touching. Talk to your partner about your feelings and concerns. Discuss any lack of desire and/or vaginal dryness with your doctor. It's an important part of your treatment and your rehabilitation. There's more to sexuality than a breast!

It is rare for a good relationship to be adversely affected by breast cancer or by a temporary lack of sexual desire. While the emotional and financial stress of the whole experience can strain a relationship, your value to your partner will probably be enhanced rather than diminished.

Most partners don't know how to approach you sexually now. They want to express their positive emotions sexually, but don't know whether or not you will be receptive, or whether sex will strain you physically. Talk about it! Develop a set of signals for each other. Explore new ways of lovemaking. Your scar may even be a new area of sexual excitement. Or, if your scar is numb (usual) or overly sensitive (unusual), you might want to shift your attention to the other breast, or another part of your body. Tell your partner. Explore together.

Above all, remember that you and your partner have been through the breast cancer ordeal together. Sexuality is one part of that process, not the whole thing. If you are patient with yourself and if you and your partner are patient with each other, this aspect of your relationship will work itself out as well.

If You're Not in a Relationship

The question that looms largest is, "When do I tell?" Generally a good rule to follow is *not right away*. Let him or her get a chance to know you as a person. After all, you are more than just a missing breast and a breast cancer survivor— don't think of yourself as damaged goods. You've climbed Mt. Everest!

When you get well past the friendship stage and are sharing confidences, that's when the time will be right. And rather than worrying that the discussion will impede a sexual relationship, you may find that it promotes one!

Helpful Hints

1) For vaginal dryness, vitamin E cream inserted into your vagina manually is sometimes recommended. Other choices are Astrolube or Replens, a lubricant inserted with a tampon-like tube that many women have found very useful.

2) If a lack of desire persists after your treatments, ask the doctor to check your testosterone level. This is a hor-

mone produced in small amounts by the ovaries that fosters libido. If it is very low, the doctor can prescribe a supplement.

3) If you're concerned about your appearance in bed, there are special bras and prostheses for sleeping. There are also inventive ways of draping nightgowns.

4) It can be helpful to get books from the library and read about sexuality. New thinking emphasizes touching, relating, talking, and sharing as important parts of sexual activity.

5) Sexual problems in breast cancer patients might be emotional rather than physical—regardless of what kind of treatment you've had. In these cases, counseling can be extremely helpful.

Notes

Chapter 29

Older Women

Older women are at greater risk for breast cancer than younger women. When the older woman is living alone, somewhat frail, and has other medical problems the situation can seem especially overwhelming. This is the time that hospital social workers, hotline volunteers, senior citizen services, your doctor, and the office or oncology nurse can be asked to help.

Assistance with home health aids, respite care for caretakers, equipment, meals, counseling and other services are often available through hotlines, the American Cancer Society, and other care giving agencies. Large print pamphlets are sometimes available for those who have trouble reading.

Just because you're in the "older woman" category, don't give up on yourself!

Older women have special problems to deal with. They are more likely to get breast cancer than younger women, but the good news is that the cancer is likely to grow more slowly.

While you may feel younger than your age, there are prejudices that you may have to fight—in other people and in society in general. Don't despair—they can be overcome.

Depending on your age and situation, some people might ask:

1) Why bother with surgery and treatments at your age?

Actually, less invasive treatments are often offered to older women. If the lesser treatment is only being offered because of your age, that is discrimination! You are entitled to the best treatment for your physical condition. Ask your doctors, "If I were twenty years younger and in the same physical condition, would this be the treatment I'd be offered?" If the answer is, "No," then ask, "Why not?"

2) Don't you know we all have to die of some thing?

Believe it or not, many people ask this insensitive question. Well, of course you know this, but aren't you entitled to as long a life as possible? Who says that a diagnosis of breast cancer is a reason to forgo potentially life-saving treatment?

Questions some older women may ask themselves include:

1) Medicare pays so little; how can I afford the treatments?

If the cost of treatment concerns you, talk to your doctor, the office nurse, or the hospital social worker. Your hotline volunteer might be able to recommend good places that accept Medicare. And many doctors, when asked, will work with you by adjusting their fees or helping you find a good referral that you can afford.

2) With my other health problems, am I not a poor candidate for the difficult treatments they use for breast cancer?

There are medical problems that older people might have. You're probably not in quite as good physical shape as you were when you were younger and you might have somewhat lower resistance to disease, which may make it harder to fight the illness. Breast cancer treatments are not given mechanically; not everyone gets the same treatment. Discuss this concern with your doctors; often they can design treatments especially suited for your physical condition.

3)   Should someone my age undergo the risks of anesthesia?

Again, discuss this with your doctor and particularly with your anesthesiologist (see chapter 16, "Preparing for Surgery"). Millions of people—from infants to people in their nineties— safely have anesthesia each year, and medical experts in anesthesia are accustomed to dealing with problems that arise. Discussing your concerns beforehand is intelligent and advised. And always insist that the answers you receive make sense to you.

Helpful Hints

1) Don't worry that Medicare only pays for screening mammograms every other year. If you've had even a suspicion of breast cancer, your mammograms are now diagnostic rather than screening, and Medicare will pay for them if your doctor so orders.

2) If you have difficulty with transportation for medical care, there are many special services offered for senior citizens. Call your local Department of Senior Citizens Affairs, your city's transportation systems, the American Cancer Society or your hotline volunteer. They will know if there are special arrangements that can be made in your area.

3) If there is no one available to care for you during recovery, ask the hospital social services center, your hotline volunteer or the doctor's nurse to arrange for a home health aide. Medicare allows for such services under certain conditions.

4) If your support system (family and friends) has shrunk—and even if it hasn't—get in touch with your hotline volunteer and ask for a referral to a support group and/or homebound counseling services.

5) Don't be ashamed if hearing or memory problems affect you. Be up front in discussing this with your treatment team. Ask them to make a note of it at the top of your chart and mention it every time you meet with them. Ask, "Did I hear you right; is that what you said?" "Please write down the directions in large print so I can read them if I forget." Put everything in your notebook, and keep your notebook in your pocketbook so you'll always know where it is. Paste a note near your telephone, reminding you where the notebook is. Also paste your doctors' numbers next to your telephone.

6) NEVER TAKE YOUR MEDICATION WITHOUT CHECKING THAT IT'S THE RIGHT ONE AND THE RIGHT DOSE. Each evening, lay out your medications for the next day. Put each medication in a separate dish and label it with the name of the medication and the time you have to take it (or "after breakfast," "before lunch," etc.). Then place the proper pills in the appropriate dish.

7) Older patients are often not as assertive as younger ones. Some feel more reluctant to ask questions or explore options. That doesn't have to be you! Remember—the more you know about your treatment and your disease and the more questions you ask, the better chance you have of getting the treatment that is best for you.

Notes

162

Chapter 30

Dealing with Insurance Problems

There are several common types of insurance problems. Here are some you might encounter. The first three are workable. The fourth can be extremely difficult or even impossible to change. In all cases, you may need legal assistance.

1) Payment for a second opinion

2) Denial of coverage for "off label use of drugs"

3) Denial of coverage for "experimental treatment"

4) Inability to change insurance companies because of a "previously existing condition"

This is what to do:

- Sometimes just a statement to your insurance company that you intend to contact a lawyer can change their decision.

- Call your breast cancer hotline and ask if there are any special legal services in your area available to breast cancer patients.

- Often a simple letter from a lawyer is enough to influence the insurance company to respond in a positive way.

- If you need a referral to a lawyer, call your local county bar association or a nearby law school. Or look in the yellow pages of the phone book under "Lawyer Referral Service."

The main questions to ask your insurance company are:

1) Will this treatment be covered?

2) What part of the payment (the co-payment) will I be responsible for?

3) What is the maximum the company will allow?

4) Is coverage provided for outpatient treatment or only inpatient treatment?

5) Is a second opinion covered? Required?

6) What about consultations?

Helpful Hints

1) Keep your insurance company informed of any changes in your life that might affect your coverage, such as marriage, divorce, loss of a job, a new job, or turning sixty-five years old.

2) Get a copy of all of your health insurance policies and make a list of company and agents' names, addresses, phone numbers, and policy numbers. Keep them all in one place.

3) With different colored pens, mark what benefits are covered and *which treatments are specifically excluded from your policy.*

4) Follow the directions in the policy carefully, i.e., preapproval, second opinion, need for special forms, etc. Add this information to your list.

5) Check with your insurance carrier before starting any treatment so that you know how they will interpret your policy.

6) When you call the company, learn the name of the insurance representative you are speaking with and, if possible, try to speak with that person each time you call. Write down the name, date, and time of your call, and all the pertinent information you get.

7) Get all agreements with your insurance company in writing. Phone agreements are not sufficient.

8) Keep copies of all the information you receive from your insurer and records of all payments that you make.

9) Most insurance companies cover the cost of a second opinion. Some require it. Check it out.

10) Ask the insurance company if they have an 800 number.

11) Ask your physician what experience s/he has had with insurance coverage for your treatment and how other patients have been able to deal with it.

12) If your insurance company allows less than you are paying for a procedure, talk to your doctor about the possibility of reducing the charges.

13) Call your breast cancer hotline and ask for guidance.

14) Be sure you have complied with the time requirements of your policy: there may be deadlines for filing or notice to be given prior to surgery.

15) Insurance companies do not generally pay for preven-

tive medicine, but they often do pay for diagnosis and treatment. Therefore, routine screening for metastases (the spread of cancer) may not be reimbursable unless there is a symptom present.

16) Assemble a list of your arguments about controversial treatments: e.g., medical journal articles supporting this treatment as appropriate for your condition (get them from toll-free 1-800-4-CANCER and/or a medical library).

17) Let the insurance company know that you are prepared to fight for the coverage.

18) Contact your state or federal legislators[1] for assistance. They have consumer advocates in their offices who can intervene. Ask your state senator for the name of a legislator on your state's insurance committee.

19) Ask a lawyer to write a letter to the insurance company indicating that you are going to press the claim.

20) If you decide to press your case, discuss with your lawyer and your hotline volunteer the issue of contacting the media (newspaper, TV, radio) to publicize your issue. There are advantages and disadvantages to this; weigh and measure them.

21) Employers must maintain preexisting insurance for the twelve weeks of unpaid leave you are entitled to under the Family and Medical Leave Act (FMLA). You are supposed to get your job back after unpaid leave.

22) If you leave your job, be sure to continue your insurance coverage under COBRA.[2]

---

1. State or federal legislators: numbers listed in the Community section of the phone book under "State" or "Federal" Governments.

2. COBRA: Consolidated Omnibus Budget Reconciliation Act. This permits employees of large companies to maintain group insurance privately after they have left a job. It's expensive.

❖ ❖ ❖

Note: If you feel you're being harassed on the job because of your illness, contact your union or state legislator[3] about your rights under the Fair Labor Standards Act Employment Bill.

If You're Uninsured

Breast cancer treatment can be very costly, but it is important that you *don't neglect yourself because of the cost.*

Note: Your local medical society and your state legislators should be made aware of the problems for people with incomes above Medicaid guidelines but without the ability to pay.

Helpful Hints

1) For information on low-cost treatment, call your local breast cancer hotline:

    Toll-free 1-800-877-8077 in New York State

    Toll-free 1-800-221-2141 in other states

    Toll-free 1-800-ACS-2345

    Or call your local hospital or medical society.

2) Talk to the hospital billing department and your physician about your financial concerns. They may be willing to make special fee arrangements or find an appropriate referral.

---

3. See chapter 31, "Individual and Community Action."

3) In requesting lowered fees from a hospital, be sure to bring with you a list of all debts including mortgage, car payments, credit card, and tuition bills.

4) If your local physician or hospital cannot arrange for you to have good, low-cost treatment, ask where it can be obtained.

5) Consider taking up temporary residence with a relative who may live in an area where low-cost treatment is available.

6) "Patient Drug Assistance Programs," run by manufacturers of the chemicals you are being given, may help with the cost of the drugs. For information, call toll-free 1-800-4-CANCER, or ask your doctor.

7) Contact your local fraternal organizations (Lions, Kiwanis, Elks) for financial assistance.

8) Agencies (such as Cancer Care in New York State) offer financial help with home health aides, etc.

9) Some states have made special arrangements with pharmaceutical companies to provide low-cost drugs for cancer therapy to low- and middle-income senior citizens who qualify. Call your state or local representatives to learn if your state has such an arrangement.

10) Look into church/synagogue assistance.

11) Tell your elected representative about your financial difficulties in paying for expensive treatments.

12) The Family and Medical Leave Act requires that qualified employees be given up to twelve weeks of unpaid leave per year for a seriously ill person or to care for an immediate family member with a serious health condition.

Notes

169

Chapter 31

Individual and Community Action

In writing this book we wanted to help women be better able to deal with all the issues of breast cancer—to be in a position to make the decisions that would be best for each individual.

For those who want to change "the system," there is a way. In fact, there are several ways. In talking to one another, one-on-one, many breast cancer patients have provided information and education that has helped them to fight this battle. In banding together with others to influence the larger system, they have inspired the government to begin to implement change.

For those who want to do more—who want to reach out to help others who are dealing with breast cancer issues or who want to try to change the system—several avenues are open.

1) *Helping others on an individual basis.* Some women find it rewarding to use their experiences to smooth the way for others. They:

> work on breast cancer hotlines, talking to people over the phone to provide information and support to those who are going through the process of a breast cancer diagnosis;

> serve as Reach to Recovery volunteers.

2) *Group and community education.* For women who enjoy meeting with people in groups, there are oppor-

tunities where professionally run programs are not available. In this case, you can:

work through a hospital to provide peer group leadership;

offer to educate community groups about the importance of early detection and second opinions;

raise money for your favorite breast cancer organization or research project.

3) *Advocacy and political action.* Those who have been through a diagnosis of breast cancer and subsequent treatment know many of the very serious issues that need to be changed in how breast cancer is dealt with in the United States. Women have banded together in towns all across the country to press for these changes. Since 1991 there has been a national organization working to bring *all* our voices together. The National Breast Cancer Coalition (NBCC) has members in each of the fifty states. The NBCC's goals are:

To increase the amount of money the government allocates to research breast cancer causes *and* a cure.

To make it possible for every woman to have equal access to *the best* breast health care.

To increase the influence and involvement of breast cancer patients in the decisions that affect their lives, including clinical trials and regulatory matters.

In the short time this organization has been in existence, it has involved individuals and grass roots groups around the country in working to increase community awareness of the unsatisfactory way in which breast cancer has been handled.

There are many problems that our institutions—both govern-
mental and medical—have failed to face in an aggressive,
appropriate, and adequate way. These include:

1) There is no known cause for breast cancer.

2) There is no known cure.

3) Early detection is not prevention.

4) Being in a "high-risk" category only explains 20–30
   percent of breast cancer cases; the other 70–80 percent are unexplained.

**The government spends a disproportionately small amount
of money on breast cancer research compared to the number
of women who get the disease—182,000 in 1993 and increasing every year.**

The incidence rate of breast cancer has risen dramatically
since the 1970s, particularly in the last decade. Today, according to the National Institutes of Health, one out of every eight
women will get breast cancer during her lifetime.

There has been essentially no change in the mortality rate
from breast cancer in the past fifty years. The percentage of
breast cancer patients who die of the disease remains the same
despite all the research on new treatments. And, in spite of the
new ways that drugs are combined, dosages intensified, and
new drugs like Taxol developed, there has been very little
change in the treatment of breast cancer in the past forty years.

Many of the treatments used for breast cancer are not covered by medical insurance because they are considered
"experimental." Some treatments considered "acceptable"
have not been adequately tested.

The list of unanswered questions and inadequate treatments goes on and on. And while it seems overwhelming, the
fact is that within eighteen months of its start the National
Breast Cancer Coalition was able to spearhead a drive for
women all around the country to tell their legislators what was

wrong—and to encourage them to begin making some significant changes.

Helpful Hints

Here are some suggestions on how to begin:

1) Call the National Breast Cancer Coalition to see where
   the nearest activist group is located. The telephone
   number is 1-202-296-7477.

2) Talk to an oncology nurse or oncology social worker in
   the hospital where you are treated for help in getting in
   touch with local advocacy groups.

3) Make an appointment to see the editor of your local
   newspaper to explain your interest and the urgent need
   to publicize this issue. Tell her or him that you can provide your own first-person experience and offer to put
   the editor in touch with others who can also provide
   information. Remember that media people are *always*
   interested in "hot," topical, and urgent matters. If the
   subject of breast cancer is not being regularly featured,
   it is because other people have made their own issues
   known and breast cancer activists have not. *Most
   media people will respect your right to privacy,* if this is
   important to you.

   Ask the editor (or feature writer or publisher) about
   the kind of help s/he can provide. Ask about the possibility of a feature or news story, or an item about want-
   ing to meet others who are as concerned about breast
   cancer as you are.

When you have a clear idea about something you think should be changed, here are some hints about how to be most effective:

1) Find out whether the issue you have is one that is handled by state legislators or by federal legislators. Research, for example, is federal; some insurance is controlled by the states, some by the federal government.

2) Research the issue. Get as many accurate facts as you can.

3) Decide *exactly* what kind of change you want. Asking for support on an issue is not as effective as asking for a yes or no vote on a particular bill. Actually, *support* is too general a word. A clear idea about exactly what it is you want to see changed, some suggestions about how it can be possible, and some reasons why it is necessary can help your congressperson know how to help you. You can find the name of the person who represents you in Congress in your phone book, in addition to the names of your U.S. senators, state senators, and assembly people.

4) Even if your legislator isn't on the committee that handles the many issues of breast cancer, s/he still represents *you* and can steer you to the right people and use his or her influence with them.

5) Be prepared with some good points (and, as you know, there are many!) to use in discussing the breast cancer issue. If s/he tells you there are "problems" with doing what you are asking, ask why. Remind her or him that this is a national epidemic—what are the priorities?

6) Don't be upset if you see an aide instead of the congressperson; aides may know more about an issue

because they are often the people who brief the legislator and suggest action. The same is true for the elected officials' secretaries. Get to know them, even if it is by telephone. They can be your most potent allies.

7) Remember that education and discussion can be more effective than confrontation. Elected officials want "hard facts." This is what they use to push through legislation.

8) Don't be afraid to tell your personal story as an example of why you are asking for a legislative change. This is a powerful strategy. Every person you will speak to has a mother, sister, lover, wife, daughter, colleague, friend. All are vulnerable to breast cancer. Remind them of this fact!

9) Follow up your visit with a thank-you note. This note should repeat your message, desires, expectations, and also your interest in making the issue of breast cancer a *front burner* priority.

10) Visit or write fairly frequently, giving additional information or asking for an update on progress on what s/he has promised to do.

11) An efficient way to do all of this is to write down the telephone numbers of your congressperson and state senator or assembly person next to your phone. Every week, on the same day and at the same hour, make those calls. Keep a record of your calls. This is what to ask:

What are you doing about the breast cancer epidemic in our country?

What have you done since we last spoke?

What have you learned since I called you on "X" date?

Good for you! Or, I haven't heard anything. What's going on?

12) Call the White House "Opinion Line" at 1-202-456-1111 and say you're concerned about breast cancer research and funding. The more often you call, the better. Your call will be relayed to the president! If you call every week, week in and week out, month in and month out, you will get a response.

You can make a difference! Thousands of women are following these guidelines already. We hope that their efforts tell you that *you are not alone!*

Notes

Resources

Hotlines

Breast Implants Hotline   Toll-free 1-800-532-4440

Cancer Fax   1-301-402-5874
                                        (faxed information about cancer)

New York Statewide
Breast Cancer Hotline   Toll-free 1-800-877-8077;
                                                              516-877-4444

Nolvadex (Tamoxifen) Patient
Assistance Program   Toll-free 1-800-424-3727

Nutritional Diet Supplements Hotline   Toll-free 1-800-776-5446

Saliva Supplements   Toll-free 1-800-968-7772

Y-ME National Breast Cancer
Organization   Toll-free 1-800-221-2141;
                                                            708-799-8228

Organizations

Breast Implant Information Network
(Command Trust Network, Inc.)
CTN, Inc.
P.O. Box 17082
Covington, KY 41047   Call Kathleen Anneken: 606-331-0055

Cancer Care, Inc.
1180 Avenue of the Americas
New York, NY 10036   212-221-3300

Chemotherapy Foundation
183 Madison Avenue
New York, NY 10016   212-213-9292

Mary-Helen Mautner Project for Lesbians with Cancer
P.O. Box 90437
Washington, DC 20002   202-332-5536

National Alliance of Breast Cancer Organizations (NABCO)
1180 Avenue of the Americas, 2nd Floor
New York, NY 10036   212-719-0154

National Coalition for Cancer Survivorship
101 Wayne Avenue, Suite 300
Silver Spring, MD 20910   301-650-8868

National Lymphedema Network
2211 Post Street, Suite 404
San Francisco, CA 94115   Toll-free 1-800-541-3259

New York City Lesbian
and Gay Health Project   212-788-4400

Reconstruction Counseling (Part of the
Einstein Medical Center's Breast
Cancer Program in Philadelphia)   Toll-free 1-800-EIN-STEIN

SAGE (Senior Action in a Gay Environment)
208 West 13th Street
New York, NY 10011   212-741-2247

YWCA Encore Program
726 Broadway
New York, NY 10003   212-614-2827

Advocacy Groups

CANACT (Cancer Patients Action Alliance)
26 College Place
Brooklyn, NY 11201   718-522-4607

The National Breast Cancer Coalition
P.O. Box 66373
Washington, DC 20035   202-296-7477

Brochures

The American Cancer Society (ACS) and the National Cancer Institute (NCI) can provide free—in several different languages—information, literature, booklets, and advice about the following subjects: mammography, biopsies, radiation, chemotherapy, breast surgery, treatment options, clinical trials, reconstructive surgery, recurrence, pain, sexuality, nutrition, and emotional support, among other things.

American Cancer Society
1599 Clifton Road, NE
Atlanta, GA 30329   Toll-free 1-800-ACS-2345

National Cancer Institute   Toll-free 1-800-4-CANCER
Alaska: toll-free 1-800-638-6070
Hawaii: call collect 808-524-1235.
Always call NCI during working hours in your time zone.

Mammography

The American College of Radiology   703-648-8900
(offers a list of mammography centers they have certified in your state)

Medical Referrals

American College of Surgeons	312-664-4050

American Society of Plastic
and Reconstructive Surgeons
444 East Algonquin Road
Arlington Heights, IL 60005   Toll-free 1-800-635-0635

The Board of Medical Specialties   Toll-free 1-800-776-2378

Second Opinion Surgical Hotline   ·Toll-free 1-800-638-6833

Strang Cancer Prevention Center   Toll-free 1-800-521-9356

To learn if your oncologist's hospital is a member of the Council of Teaching Hospitals of the American Medical Colleges, write to:

Hospital Inquiries
Division of Clinical Services
Association of Medical Colleges
2450 N Street, NW
Washington, DC 20037

Clinical Trials

Community Clinical Oncology Program (CCOP) (July 1991; updated periodically). This is a list of the 129 community programs in 31 states that have been selected by the National Cancer Institute to participate in the introduction of the newest clinical protocols and to accrue patients to clinical trials.

Autologous Bone Marrow Transplantation: Facing the Challenge NABCO (see Advocacy Groups above). 22-minute video. 212-719-0154.

Susan K. Stewart. *Bone Marrow Transplants Newsletter,* 1992. Write to: *BMT Newsletter,* 1985 Spruce Avenue, Highland Park, IL 60035. 708-831-1913.

Nontraditional Treatments

We suggest that these be considered *in addition to,* not in place of traditional treatments.

The American Cancer Society
*Unproven Methods of
Cancer Management* (1991)   Toll-free 1-800-ACS-2345

CANHELP
3111 Paradise Bay Road
Port Ludlow, WA 98365-9771   206-437-2291
Conducts worldwide search of alternative options for cancer treatment. $400.00

FACT (Foundation for Alternative
  Cancer Therapies)
Box 1242, Old Chelsea Station
New York, NY 10113   212-741-2790

FAIM (Foundation for the Advancement
  of Innovative Medicine)
2 Executive Boulevard, Suite 204
Suffern, NY 10901   914-368-9797

The National Council Against
  Health Fraud   Toll-free 1-800-821-6671
Or write to Consumer Health Information Research Institute
3521 Broadway
Kansas City, MO 64111

Unconventional Cancer Treatments (Summary, OTA-H-406, $1.75, September 1990). Order from:
U.S. Government Printing Office
Washington, DC 20402-9325   202-783-3238
For the summary, refer to GPO Stock Number 052-003-0128-1.

Alternatives for the Health Conscious Individual (newsletter)
Mountain Home Publishing
P.O. Box 829
Ingram, TX 78025
Editor: Dr. David G. Williams

Dr. I. William Lane and Linda Comac. *Sharks Don't Get Cancer.* Garden City, N.Y.: Avery Publishing Group, 1992.

Ralph Moss, Ph.D., *Cancer Therapy: The Independent Consumer's Guide to Non-Toxic Treatment and Prevention.* New York: Equinox Press, 1992.

Michael Lerner, Ph.D., Rachel Naomi Remen, M.D.
Commonweal (Weeklong residential cancer help program; includes yoga, meditation, diet, art therapy, etc.)
P.O. Box 316
Bolinas, CA 94924   415-868-0970

Newsletters/Subscriptions

National Alliance of Breast Cancer Organizations (NABCO)
1180 Avenue of the Americas, 2nd Floor
New York, NY 10036   212-719-0154

The National Women's Health Network
(Women's Health Information Service)
1325 G Street, NW
Washington, DC 20005   202-347-1140

Sexual Counseling Referrals (Nationwide)

Helen Singer Kaplan, M.D.
30 East 76th Street
New York, NY 10021   212-249-2914

Exercise

The YWCA Encore Program National Headquarters
726 Broadway
New York, NY 10003   212-614-2827

Wigs and Prostheses

Jacques Darcel   Toll-free 1-800-445-1897

Y-ME Prosthesis and Wig Bank   Toll-free 1-800-221-2141

Buyer's Guide to Wigs and Hairpieces
Ruth Weintraub Co., Inc.
420 Madison Avenue, Suite 406
New York, NY 10017   212-838-1333

Edith Imre Foundation for Loss of Hair
30 West 57th Street
New York, NY 10019   212-757-8160

Jean Paree Corp.
555 South 2nd East
Salt Lake City, UT 84111   Toll-free 1-800-422-9447

Fashion Wigs by Paula Young
21 Bristol Drive
South Easton, MA 02375

Jacquelyn International Fashion Products, Inc.
Dept. C, 15 West 37th Street
New York, NY 10018   Toll-free 1-800-272-2424

Flex-Pads International
(Soft tissue prostheses)
Isabel Mandelkern, President
8833 West 75th Street
Overland Park, KS 66204   Toll-free 1-800-527-5275;
                                                      913-649-2525

Appearance

Look Good . . . Feel Better
Call toll-free 1-800-395-LOOK or your local ACS office

Insurance

Cancer Treatments Your Insurance Should Cover (March 1991).
Order from:
Association of Community Cancer Centers
11600 Nebel Street, Suite 201
Rockville, MD 20852   301-984-9496

National Insurance Consumer Helpline   Toll-free 1-800-942-4242

Equal Employment Opportunity Commission "Technical Assistance
  Manual"
1801 L Street, NW
Washington, DC 20507   Toll-free: 1-800-669-3362

Environment

Environmental Protection Agency
Public Information Center
401 M Street, SW
Washington, DC 20460   202-260 2080
(Provides information on ridding your home of known carcinogens.)

Computer Programs

Here are some numbers that may come in handy:

CompuServe: Toll-free 1-800-848-8199
Medline: Toll-free 1-800-478-1126
Grateful Med: Toll-free 1-800-638-8480

The American Self-Help Clearinghouse tracks 700 health-related topics and publishes the *Self-Help Sourcebook* for $10.00. 201-625-7101.

The Health Resource Inc. will run Medline searches for you, including information about holistic and alternative therapies. The cost is from $85.00 to $175.00 and they return your money if you're not satisfied. 501-329-5272.

Death and Dying

National Hemlock Society
Box 11830
Eugene, OR 97440
(Group that discusses the issue of suicide.)

Choice in Dying
200 Varick Street
New York, NY 10014   Toll-free 1-800-989-WILL
(Nonprofit organization that provides information about a living will
and power of attorney for health-care decisions, and maintains a
registry for them.)

Bibliography

Recommended

Susan M. Love, M.D., *Dr. Susan Love's Breast Book*. New York: Addison-Wesley Publishing Company, Inc., 1990 (paperback).

Personal Stories

Judith Glassman, *The Cancer Survivors and How They Did It*. New York: The Dial Press, 1983.

Deborah H. Kahane, *No Less a Woman: Ten Women Shatter the Myths About Breast Cancer*. New York: Prentice Hall Press, 1990.

Ronnie Kaye, *Spinning Straw into Gold: Your Emotional Recovery from Breast Cancer*. New York: Fireside/Simon & Schuster, 1991.

Lawrence LeShan, *Cancer as a Turning Point*. New York: Dutton, 1989.

Andy Murcia and Bob Stewart's story, *Man to Man: When the Woman You Love Has Breast Cancer*, is written from the husbands' point of view. New York: St. Martins Press, 1989.

Betty Rollins, *First You Cry*. New York: Harper & Row, 1986.

Self-Help

Annette and Richard Bloch, *Guide for Cancer Supporters*. Kansas City, Mo.: R. A. Bloch Cancer Foundation Inc., 1992.

Pat Brack with Ben Brack, *Moms Don't Get Sick*. Melices Publishing, 1990.

Nancy Bruning, *Coping with Chemotherapy*. New York: Ballantine Books, 1985 (paperback).

Nancy Bruning, *Breast Implants: Everything You Need to Know*. Alameda, Calif.: Hunter House, 1992 (paperback).

Deepak Chopra, M.D., *Quantum Healing*. New York: Bantam Books, 1989.

Norman Cousins, *Anatomy of an Illness*. New York: Bantam Books, 1986.

Lawrence LeShan, *You Can Fight for Your Life*. New York: M. Evans, 1977.

Carolyn Stearns Parkinson, *My Mommy Has Cancer*. Park Press, P.O. Box 23205, Rochester, NY 14692-3205.

Wendy Williams, *The Power Within*. New York: HarperCollins, 1990.

Guided Imagery

Jeanne Achterberg, *Imagery in Healing*. Boston: New Science Library, Shambhala, 1985.

Shakti Gawain, *Creative Visualization*. San Rafael, Calif.: New World Library, 1978.

Bernie Siegel, *Love, Medicine & Miracles*. New York: Harper & Row, 1986.

O. Carl Simonton and Stephanie Simonton, *Getting Well Again*. Los Angeles: J. P. Tarcher, 1978.

Periodicals

Coping: Living with Cancer
2019 Carothers
Franklin, TN 37064   615-790-7553
(Quarterly magazine for cancer survivors.)

Natural Health: The Guide to Well-Being
17 Station Street
P.O. Box 1200
Brookline Village, MA 02147-9902   Toll-free 1-800-635-0100
(Monthly magazine featuring traditional and alternative health strategies.)

Sexuality

Sexuality and Cancer: For the Woman Who Has Cancer, and Her Partner (Pamphlet, 1988 edition)   ACS: toll-free 1-800-ACS-2345

Linda Dackman, *Up Front: Sex and the Post-Mastectomy Woman.* New York: Penguin Books, 1990.

Helen Singer Kaplan, "A neglected issue: The sexual side effects of current therapies for breast cancer." *Journal of Sex and Marital Therapy,* vol. 18, no. 1, Spring 1992.

Nutrition

Saundra N. Aker, and Polly Lennsen, *A Guide to Good Nutrition During and After Chemotherapy and Radiation* (3rd edition, 1988, $6.00). Order from The Fred Hutchinson Cancer Research Center Clinical Nutrition Program, 206-667-4834.

Kedar N. Prasad, *Vitamins Against Cancer.* Healing Arts Press, 1 Park Street, Rochester, VT 05767 (1989, $6.95).

The Diet Your Doctor Won't Give You. Published by the National Women's Health Network. Contact NWHN, 1325 G Street, NW, Washington, DC 20005; 202-347-1140 (1987, $1.00, pamphlet).

Ruth Spear, *Low Fat and Loving It.* New York: Warner Books, 1991 (paperback).

Tamoxifen

Valerie J. Wieve, and Michael De Gregorio, *A Guide to Understanding Tamoxifen.* New Haven, Conn.: Yale University Press, 1993.

Implants

Silicone Implants (a bibliography)
to order: GPO #817-008-00006-4
Department of Documents
Box 371904
Pittsburgh, PA 15250-7954

Order documents about silicone and breast implants from:

Food & Drug Administration
Freedom of Information Staff (HFI-35)
5600 Fishers Lane
Rockville, MD 20857 Toll-free 1-800-532-4440

ASIS (American Silicone Implant Survivors)
1288 Cork Elm Drive
Kirkwood, MO 63122 314-821-0115

Appendix A

How to Create a Notebook

Size. Your notebook should be easy to carry.

Type. A looseleaf notebook lets you add pages as you need them. A spiral notebook can open flat.

Format. On the **first page** of your notebook, write your doctor's number and the name and number of your hotline volunteer. Also, write "return to" with your name, address and phone number, in case the notebook gets lost.

On the **second page** write down your relevant medical history—symptoms and dates, treatments and dates. Leave a few **empty pages** so you can add to this.

Next are pages to keep track of **contacts** you make and information you get on the phone or during doctors' visits.

A format that's easy to remember and designed to yield the most information is the journalist's format, which asks *who, when, where, why, what,* and *how.* It may not seem necessary to fill in every category, but later on, when you have dozens of referrals, the information will come in handy and will let you sort out who said what and when and why.

This is how you may want to design your notebook:

WHO: Here you can put the name of the person you speak to: your doctor, the office staff person, a friend, etc. In short, any resource. Include the person's title, if any, since you may have to write to him or her in the future, or you may recommend this person to a friend. Also include WHO recommended this person.

WHEN: *Always put the date* and even the time of day (so you remember the order in which things happened).

WHERE: Write down where you can contact or see the person. If you are doing book research, write down the library. Similarly, it could be a doctor's office, laboratory, or a telephone conversation. Try to put down all the information, including the zip code and fax number, since you may use this resource later. Also, leave room for directions to the place.

WHY: State the purpose of your contacts and, again, who referred you.

WHAT: *What* you are asking. Leave a lot of room for this section to include all of your questions.

HOW: *How* the person responds; the answers you receive. In this section, you can include subjects like directions for taking medications or undergoing tests, or any referral the person may give you.

On the **back page** start writing questions that you think of. As you record the answers, cross off the questions.

Here is how a typical entry might look:

WHO: Talked to Dr. Marcia Smith, radiologist (recommended by Jane S. who used her).

WHEN: Wednesday, December 9, 1992, at 10:30 A.M.

WHERE: 123 Main Street, Suite 100, Anywhere, Any State,
             12345.

Phone: 203-123-4567.

Direction: Take Post Road to first intersection. Make right at
             light onto Main Street and go three blocks to red
             brick building on right, #123. Room 306. Elevator
             in back. Park on street: 25 cents per hour.

WHY: Her specialty is postlumpectomy. Jane says easy
             to talk to.

WHAT: Is outcome as good as mastectomy?

             Why is lumpectomy advantageous?

             What will follow-up treatments be? Time of day?
             Number of weeks?

             Does insurance cover treatments?

             Is there parking near her office?

HOW: Encouraged lumpectomy and lymph nodes as bet-
             ter. Mastectomy not necessary. Radiation 5 times
             per week, open from 6 A.M. to 8 P.M. Insurance plus
             co-payment. Meter parking (quarters). Need mam-
             mography films. Insurance forms. Good feeling
             about her. Knows Dr. A.

Appendix B

How to Become Your Own Investigative Reporter
(And Find Out What You Need to Know)

One of the greatest causes of anxiety is *not knowing*. Just when you need to find out someone's name, the side effects of a medication, where to find a clinical trial, how to look up information, or any of the million questions you're presented with, it all seems "too much."

Yet it's very doable! And it all starts with the right attitude. Before you seek an answer, tell yourself two things:

1) This information is available.

2) I can find it.

From this point on, it becomes easier and easier. First, write down exactly what you want to know. For instance, What are the side effects of Tamoxifen? Then take time out to tell yourself what you *already know* about Tamoxifen. You know that it's a drug. You know that the library has books and articles about drugs. You know that the pharmacist has information about drugs. You know that many computer programs have information about drugs. If you have the original bottle, you know the manufacturer.

So, without knowing Tamoxifen's side effects, you already know a lot! And much information can be gotten over the telephone. In this case, you can go to (or call) your local library and ask the librarian if s/he has a book or article that can tell you the information you're seeking. Pharmacists have printouts of medication effects; they are available to you. Your breast cancer hotline also has information to tell you, and booklets to mail you.

The telephone can be your best ally. To find out the information you want over the telephone, follow these simple rules:

1) Write down beforehand the questions you want to ask. It's easy to forget everything you want to know, especially when calling about a subject that is unfamiliar to you, and in a time of stress.

2) Always have a pen and paper handy to write down the information you're receiving. Don't waste your own or the other person's time while you look for a pen or paper.

3) Ask to whom you're speaking. Don't forget to write down his or her name. Often the operator or secretary can be your best ally and either get you to the right resource or refer you to another source.

4) Be direct. When you call, identify yourself and say what you're calling about immediately. For instance, "Hello, my name is Jane Smith. I have breast cancer and I want to find out about [Tamoxifen, lumpectomy, clinical trials, prostheses, etc.]." Before going into details, ask, "Have I called the right place?"

5) If you're going to be switched to someone else, ask for that extension number first, so you can call back directly if you are accidentally cut off.

6) Try to stick to the main purpose of your call: your specific question(s). You may be tempted to go into detail,

but if the person you've called has to get off the phone quickly, your question may not be answered.

7) Keep a record. If you are making many calls about different subjects, get some folders and label them (for instance, "Tamoxifen," "Lumpectomy," "Wigs," etc.). Keep the files in one place (preferably a box that can be found easily). Over the course of your experience, you may find articles of interest and help that you want to add. Then when you want the information, it's right at your fingertips.

8) Some people don't mind if you use a tape recorder. There are also devices that allow you to record someone over the phone. The rule here is: Ask first! If you say, "I'd like to record what you have to say so I am sure that I am hearing and understanding it accurately," more often than not the person on the phone is agreeable. If not, assure them that the call will *not* be taped.

9) If you have an appointment to see someone from whom you are seeking information, write down your questions beforehand. Discuss this appointment with your hotline volunteer, a friend, or family member, to get ideas for additional questions. Again, write them down.

10) Thank the person you're speaking with—s/he will appreciate this nicety and, if you have to call back, may remember you!

11) If you have access to a computer, you can buy a software package that will give you medical information—like CompuServe, Medline, Grateful Med, and others. See Resources.

Appendix C
Mammography Guidelines

At any age, if you have cystic breasts, a family history of breast cancer, or are symptomatic, discuss a schedule of mammography with your doctor. Around age thirty-five or forty get a baseline screening mammogram. Starting at age fifty get a mammogram every year.

Between ages thirty-five and fifty each woman should make her own decision, after discussion with her doctor and a review of the controversy. There has been some question as to whether or not women younger than fifty should get mammograms. Before forty, and in some women before fifty, breast tissue is too dense for tumors to be seen on mammograms.

When there is a history of breast cancer in the family, some doctors believe that the early detection mammography offers can be life-saving. Women under fifty who have had tumors discovered by mammography believe the procedure saved their lives.

Appendix D

Breast Self-Examination (BSE)

Most women (or their lovers) discover their own breast lumps. In our experience, it is not uncommon for a woman to have a screening mammogram that shows nothing, but to discover shortly afterward that she has a lump in her breast.

Many physicians and health educators recommend that women practice monthly breast self-examination as a part of early detection practices. Monthly BSE helps a woman be more conscious of her breasts and the need for the other two important parts of an early detection program: annual physician examination and mammography (see appendix C). However, this may be a false security since there is no clinical evidence that practicing BSE has any impact on breast cancer mortality. Self-discovered lumps are usually found accidentally—in the shower, while getting dressed, or during sex play—and not while practicing BSE. However, any woman who has found a lump through BSE believes strongly in its effectiveness.

For these women who are interested, here is what to do.

Examine your lumpectomy or mastectomy scar and look for any signs of redness, thickening, or hardness. Also, report any pain in your shoulder, hip, lower back, or pelvis to your doctor.

If you want to practice BSE, go to a nurse practitioner or doctor to learn how to do it. When you are taught to distinguish between the "normal" lumpiness of cystic breasts and other masses, you may still feel a lump and not be sure about it. When in doubt, have your doctor check it out.

Directions for BSE

For women who get regular periods, the best time to examine your breasts is about a week after your period. If you do not get regular periods, then do it on the same day of each month.

- *In the shower:* Hands glide easily over wet skin. With flat fingers, move with a gentle motion over each part of your breast and under your arms. Use the right hand to examine the left breast and the left hand to examine the right breast. Check for any lump, hard knot, or thickening. Feel under the arms as well, where your lymph nodes are.

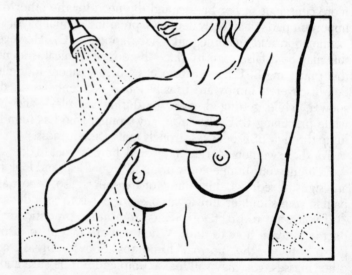

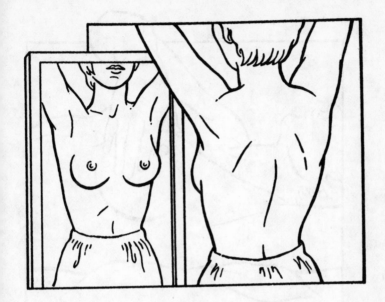

- *In front of a mirror:* Stand with your arms at your side and then raise them both over your head. Look for any changes in the contour of each breast, a swelling, a dimpling of the skin, or any changes in the nipples.

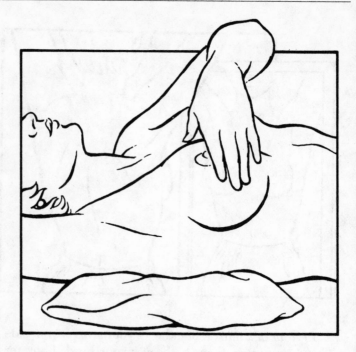

- *Lying down:* Place a pillow under your shoulder on the same side as the breast you are examining. Place the arm on that side behind your head. Then use the top third of the fingers on your hand to feel for lumps or thickening. Press firmly enough to know how your breast feels. Move around each breast in the same way every time; either (a) in a circular motion, (b) up and down, or (c) in wedgelike segments.

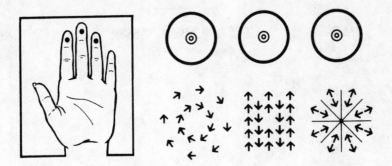

- Finally, squeeze the nipple of each breast gently between your thumb and index finger.

- If you see or feel any changes in your breasts or if you note any discharge from your nipple, see your doctor right away.

Record questionable areas you find during BSE here.

DATE	LEFT OR RIGHT BREAST	SECTION

Chemotherapy Drugs and Some of Their Possible Side Effects

These are only POSSIBLE side effects.

Do not let this list scare you into rejecting chemotherapy.

Not every breast cancer patient will experience these side effects. Discuss the possibilities with your doctor.

This is not intended as a definitive list of all chemotherapies and all side effects. We have included these so that those who want to can check a particular symptom and verify whether or not it might be due to a side effect.

In all cases we suggest you report any side effect to your doctor, and discuss it further with him or her.

Altretamine (HMM, Hexalen, HXM, NSC #13875)

Nausea, vomiting, abdominal cramps, anorexia, diarrhea. Low white blood count, low platelets. Tingling sensations, sensitivity to touch, exaggerated reflexes, motor weakness, decreased sensory sensations, decreased sensation of touch, agitation, hallucinations, confusion, lethargy, depression, coma. Weight loss.

Aminoglutethimide (Cytadren, Elipten, BA-16038)

Low white blood cell count, absence of some white blood cells, low count of all blood cells. Reddening and raised eruption of the skin occasionally associated with fever. Pustular psoriasis, loss of skin surface, mouth sores. Stomach aches. Lassitude and fatigue. Unsteady gait, dizziness, rapid eyeball movements, drowsiness. Adrenal insufficiency. Sudden drop in blood pressure and low blood salt levels (due to decreased aldosterone secretion). Masculinization, muscle ache, fever. Rarely: hypothyroidism; a systemic syndrome resembling lupus; jaundice; elevated liver enzymes. Possible elevated serum cholesterol levels in patients with breast cancer, which may predispose to atherosclerosis; great variation in levels between patients, returning to normal level within a few weeks after therapy is stopped.

Carmustine (BCNU, BiCNU, bis-Chloronitrosourea)

Low white blood count and blood clotting problems occur within two to thirty-five days and may last sixty days; they may be cumulative. Nausea and vomiting. Reversible toxicity from elevated liver enzymes. Clouding of lung tissue, especially with prolonged therapy and higher doses. It has been recommended that a cumulative dose of 1400 mg/m^2 should not be exceeded. Low blood pressure (from rapid or concentrated infusion). Decrease in kidney size and renal failure with large doses. Burning at injection site and along vein; facial flushing, dizziness.

Chlorambucil (Leukeran)

Low white blood count and blood clotting problems, dose-related. Cumulative, dose-limiting suppression of bone marrow has been observed in some patients; anemia. Loss of hair (uncommon), dermatitis (rare), itching (rare). Nausea, vomiting, and anorexia are relatively uncommon. Reduced lung capacity (rare). Sterility (amenorrhea, low sperm production), possible secondary malignancy (i.e., leukemia), cystitis, damage of nerves going to the extremities.

Cisplatin (Platinol, CDDP, DDP, DACP, cis-Platinum, Platinum)

Low white blood count and blood clotting problems occur, but are rarely dose-limiting; anemia. Hair loss (uncommon). Nausea and vomiting are common and may persist for twenty-four to ninety-six hours; anorexia. Kidney toxicity is dose-related and relatively uncommon with adequate fluid intake and urine production. Elevated liver enzymes. Nerve damage in extremities (parasthesias), common and dose-limiting when the cumulative cisplatin dose exceeds 400 mg/m². Seizures (rare). Ear problems manifested initially by high-frequency hearing loss; dizziness (uncommon); muscle spasms caused by low blood level of magnesium. Low blood levels of calcium and salt. Vein irritation, optic disc swelling (rare), severe allergic reactions (rare), fatigue.

Cyclophosphamide (Cytoxan, CTX, CPM, Neosar)

Low white blood count; lowest about nine to fourteen days after administration and recovery in eighteen to twenty-five days; spares platelets. Hair loss. Nausea and vomiting (begins six to ten hours after administration). Increased liver enzymes. Headache, dizziness. Interstitial thickening of lung tissue (rare). Heart damage. Bloody urine (onset of cystitis may be delayed from twenty-four hours to several weeks). Metallic taste during injection; nasal congestion; testicular atrophy, amenorrhea; may be long-term. Rarely fatal reactions. Harmful to fetus. May cause secondary cancers.

Dactinomycin (Actinomycin-D, ACT-D, Actinomycin-C, Cosmegen)

Low platelet and leukocyte counts that occur approximately three weeks after treatment. Acnelike rashes, skin blotches. Abnormal heartbeat. Hair loss. Nausea and vomiting (often worsening with successive daily doses), occurring about one hour after a dose and lasting several hours; trouble swallowing, inflammation of the rectum, and diarrhea. Fluid retention in the abdomen. Enlarged liver, hepatitis. Other: "Radiation recall" (skin irritation or even tissue death in previously irradiated areas); low blood calcium. Secondary cancers.

Dexamethasone (Daunomycin, Rubidomycin, Cerubidine)

Low white blood cell count reaching lowest levels between one and two weeks after beginning treatment. Rash; hair loss, blood clots or local tissue death if drug leaks out of IV tubing. Nausea, vomiting, commonly occurring one hour after a dose and lasting for several hours; diarrhea, mouth irritation. Irregular heartbeat, usually transient; congestive heart damage; maximum total (lifetime) dose of 500–600mg/m^2 is recommended because of cumulative toxic effects on the heart. Red urine, but not blood in the urine. Transient fever. Elevations in enzymes.

Doxorubicin (Adriamycin, Rubex, ADR)

Low white blood cell count (dose-limiting). Low platelets and anemia; nadir reached in ten to fourteen days; recovery in twenty-one days. Hair loss, usually complete. Discoloration of the skin. Radiation recall. Nausea and vomiting, sometimes severe; anorexia, diarrhea; inflammation of mucous membranes, especially with daily-times-three schedule. Irregular heartbeat; electrocardiogram changes; rare sudden death. Congestive heart failure due to total cumulative dose; risk is greater with total doses greater than 550mg/m^2, chest irradiation, preexisting cardiac disease, advanced age; risk is reduced with weekly or continuous infusion regimens. Other: Red discoloration of urine; fever; anaphylactoid reaction; possibly cystitis or liver toxicity. Local reactions: flushing along vein; facial flush.

Floxuridine (FUDR, 5-FUDR)

Low white blood cell count; less commonly blood clotting problems, dose- and schedule-related; more common with bolus dose regimens; anemia. Hair loss, generally mild; dermatitis; localized reddening of the skin; rash, pigmentation changes, itching, scratching—all rare. Nausea, vomiting, anorexia; diarrhea, more common with continuous infusion; inflammation of mucous membranes, dose-related, more common with continuous infusions; gastritis; inflammation of intestines; duodenal ulcer. Increased liver enzymes. Hardening of the bile duct (sclerosis); jaundice; inflammation of the gall bladder; cirrhosis (rare); mild and transient with intravenous injection, but dose-limiting with intra-arterial infusion to the liver. Rarely, unsteady gait, blurred vision, fatigue, headache, depression, vertigo, rapid eyeball movements, seizures, partial paralysis. Other: rarely, fever, painful urination, hiccups, excessive tearing from the eyes, lethargy, malaise, weakness.

Fluorouracil (5-FU, Adrucil, Efudex)

Low white blood cell count; anemia; can be dose-limiting; less common with continuous infusion. Dermatitis, nail changes, hyperpigmentation, hand-foot syndrome with protracted infusions, hair loss. Nausea, vomiting, anorexia; diarrhea, can be dose-limiting; inflammation of mucous membranes, more common with five-day infusion, occasionally dose-limiting; severe, choleralike diarrhea that can be fatal when given with leucovorin. Headache and unsteady gait. Angina, noted with continuous infusion. Eye irritation, nasal discharge, watering of eyes, blurred vision. Hepatitis with liver infusion.

Fluoxymesterone (Halotestin, Ora-testryl, FLU)

High blood level of calcium, especially in immobilized patients with bone disease. Swelling due to sodium retention. Liver function abnormalities, usually reversible when drug is discontinued. Masculinization in the female, with increased facial hair, clitoral enlargement, increased libido, and voice deepening. Enlargement of the breasts occurs in some men at high doses. Patchy hair loss; acne. Bone marrow stimulation, may be useful in patients with marrow-suppressive disease.

Gosrelin (Zoladex)

Local discomfort occasionally lasting up to thirty minutes; rarely, local rash, perhaps due to local anesthetic; rarely, other rashes. Infrequent nausea, vomiting, diarrhea, constipation. Elevated serum cholesterol. Hot flashes, decreased libido, enlargement of breasts in males; cessation of period and spotting in females. Tumor flare, consisting of increased bone pain. Urinary retention or spinal cord compression may occur in up to 20 percent of patients in the first two weeks of treat-

ment; blocked by antiandrogens (flutamide). Other: Tumor of
the pituitary gland has been reported in rats; depression rare.

Ifofamide (Ifex, Mitoxan, Holoxan, Naxamide)

Low white blood cell counts, low platelet count (dose-limiting); anemia. Nausea, vomiting, anorexia, constipation, diarrhea, salivation, inflammation of tongue. Hair loss, rash, hives.
Elevated liver enzymes, anemia. Bleeding, cystitis (incidence
related to dose and schedule; more common with a single high
dose); elevated creatinine. Sleepiness, lethargy, disorientation,
confusion, dizziness, malaise. Other: low serum salt and potassium, phlebitis, fever, high or low blood pressure.

Leucovorin (Wellcovorin, Folinic Acid, LV, LCV)

Increased platelet count. Skin rash, hives, itching. Nausea,
upset stomach, diarrhea. Wheezing (possibly allergic in ori-
gin). Other: headache; may potentiate the toxic effects of flu-
oropyrimidine therapy, resulting in increased blood and gastrointestinal symptoms (diarrhea, inflammed tongue).

Leuprolide (Leupron, Leuprorelin Acetate)

Hot flashes (in about 50 percent of patients), impotence,
enlarged breasts in men, breast tenderness, decrease in libido,
decreased testicular size. EKG changes, reduced blood supply
to tissues, high blood pressure, peripheral swelling; thrombo-
sis/phlebitis, irregular heartbeats, heart attack, low blood pressure, pulmonary embolus, stroke—all uncommon. Insomnia,
sleep disturbance; uncommonly, tingling sensations, anxiety,

blurred vision, lethargy, memory disorder, mood swings, nervousness, numbness, hearing disorder, light-headed feeling/blackouts. Anorexia, nausea, constipation, taste change, diarrhea. Dermatitis, local skin reaction, hair growth or loss, itching, pigment changes, other lesions. Other: tumor flare, manifested as increased pain at tumor sites, sometimes causing spinal cord compression or urinary retention; muscle aches, weakness, anemia, urinary tract symptoms.

Lomustine (CCNU, CeeNU)

Suppression of bone marrow function (leukopenia and low platelet count) is expected, dose-limiting and cumulative. Anemia occurs less frequently and is cumulative. Hair loss—uncommon and usually mild. Nausea, vomiting, and anorexia occur occasionally; they usually begin forty-five minutes to six hours after administration. Anorexia may persist for two to three days after nausea and vomiting have subsided. Inflammation of mucous membranes is uncommon. Elevated liver enzymes. Kidney dysfunction (increased serum creatinine, decreased creatinine clearance) is uncommon and related to the cumulative dose. With long-term administration, pulmonary dysfunction (shortness of breath, decreased diffusing capacity, thickening of tissue) can occur. Disorientation, lethargy, unsteady gait, and speech problems. Other: fatigue, pallor, menstrual cycle irregularities (amenorrhea), second malignancy (leukemia).

Mechlorethamine (HN₂, Mustargen, Nitrogen Mustard)

Suppression of bone marrow, clots in veins. Discoloration of infused vein, hair loss; use of the antidote sodium thiosulfate is indicated if IV solution leaks onto skin. Nausea, vomiting, diarrhea. Other: metallic taste, amenorrhea, impaired sperm production.

Medroxyprogesterone (Provera, Depo-Provera, Amen, Curretab, Cycrin)

Menstrual changes, amenorrhea, enlarged breasts, lactation, hot or cold flashes. Nausea, jaundice, weight gain (or loss). Hypersensitivity, hives, itching, allergic swelling, generalized rash, fatal reaction. Hair loss, acne, excessive hairiness, residual lump, discoloration of skin, or sterile abcesses at site of injection. Nervousness, insomnia, somnolence, fatigue, dizziness, depression. Retention of fluid, clots in veins, pulmonary embolism.

Megestrol (Megace, Megestrol Acetate)

Nausea, vomiting, abdominal pain—all uncommon; diarrhea and constipation have been reported with high doses. Vaginal bleeding or discharge; menstrual changes (menstrual irregularities). Hair loss (uncommon). Headache; carpal tunnel syndrome. Hot flashes, clots in veins, embolism; fluid retention, edema; hypertension with high doses. High blood calcium with high doses; irreversible insulin-dependent diabetes mellitus developed in a woman six weeks after initiation of megestrol acetate, 160 mg/day. Other: rapid breathing; weight gain and increased appetite; megestrol may be unsafe in patients with breakdown of blood pigment.

Melphalan (L-PAM, Alkeran, L-Phenylalanine Mustard, L-Sarcolysin)

Suppression of bone marrow function (low white blood cell count, low platelet count), which can be cumulative; recovery can be prolonged (six to eight weeks). Itching, dermatitis, rash. Nausea, vomiting (rare). Hypersensitivity: hives, itching, rash, fatal reaction rare.

Methotrexate (MTX, Mexate-AQ, Folex, Folex PFS, Abitrexate, Rheumatrex, Amethopterin)

Low white blood cell count, low platelet count; dose-related, more likely with prolonged drug exposure; anemia. Skin redness and/or rash, sometimes itchy; hair loss; sensitivity to light; boil formation; loss of skin pigment or hyperpigmentation; acne; spider veins; skin peeling and cystlike skin eruptions; inflammation of hair follicles. Nausea and vomiting, uncommon with conventional doses and usually mild; inflammation of tongue common, dose- and infusion-duration-related and highly variable; diarrhea; anorexia; vomiting of blood, blood in the stools. Renal dysfunction: dose-related, more likely to occur in patients with already compromised renal function, dehydration, or on other nephrotoxic drugs, manifested by increased creatinine and blood in the urine. Increased liver enzymes; hepatic fibrosis and cirrhosis, more likely to occur in patients receiving long-term continuous or daily methotrexate treatment. Damage to brain tissue, more commonly with multiple doses into the cerebrospinal fluid and in patients who have received cranial irradiation; tiredness, weakness, confusion, unsteady gait, tremors, irritability, seizures, coma. Acute side effects of methotrexate given into the cerebrospinal fluid may include dizziness, blurred vision, headache, back pain, neck rigidity, seizures, paralysis, partial paralysis. Allergic: fever and chills, rash, hives, and fatal reaction. Ocular: conjunctivitis; excessive eye tearing; cortical blindness has occurred with high doses. Pulmonary: inflammation of the lungs, thickening of lung tissue, cough, dyspnea. Other: malaise; osteoporosis; high uric acid count; reversible diminished production of sperm cells.

Mitomycin (Mutamycin, Mitomycin C)

Low white blood cell count, low platelet count; late, cumulative and dose-limiting anemia; renal failure, very low white blood cell count, pulmonary edema, and hypotension rare. Inflammation of tongue, hair loss, dermatitis, itching; death of tissues, ulceration and cellulitis if infusion goes outside of tubing under skin; skin redness and ulceration weeks to months after administration and distant from the site of injection. Abdominal pain, enlarged liver and liver failure in patients receiving mitomycin and autologous bone marrow transplantation. Tingling sensations. Interstitial inflammation of the lungs (infrequent but severe); acute bronchospasm. Kidney toxicity, increasing in frequency when doses exceed 50mg/m^2), manifested as increased serum creatinine and BUN (blood urea nitrogen). Other: fatigue, pain on injection, phlebitis, fever, lethargy, weakness, blurred vision.

Mitoxantrone (Novantrone, DHAD, DHAQ)

Low white blood cell count, low platelet count, anemia. Hair loss (mild), itching, dry skin. Nausea and vomiting (usually preventable); diarrhea, inflammation of mucous membranes, abdominal pain. Congestive heart failure; irregular heartbeats; rapid heartbeats; chest pain. Low blood pressure. Hives, rash. Transient increase in liver enzymes; jaundice (rare); hyperbilirubinemia. Headache; seizures (rare). Cough, shortness of breath. Other: blue discoloration of the whites of the eyes, veins; blue discoloration of the urine and stool, may persist for twenty-four to forty-eight hours after administration; fever; conjunctivitis; phlebitis; amenorrhea; tissue ulceration and necrosis if infusion leaks under skin (rare).

Prednisone (Deltasone, Orasone, Medicortone, Panasol-S, Liquid-Pred)

Increased white blood cell count. Nausea, vomiting, anorexia; increased appetite and weight gain; peptic ulceration. Rash; skin atrophy; facial hair growth, acne, facial redness, leaking blood under the skin (usually from injection site). Menstrual changes (amenorrhea, menstrual irregularities). Insomnia; muscle weakness; euphoria, psychosis, depression; headache, vertigo, seizures. Fluid retention and edema; hypertension; high potassium levels. Cataracts; increased intraocular pressure; protrusion of eyeballs. Low blood sugar; decreased glucose tolerance; aggravation or precipitation of diabetes mellitus; adrenal suppression. Other: osteoporosis (and resulting back pain); serious infections, including herpes zoster, varicella zoster, fungal infections, *Pneumocystis carinii*, tuberculosis; muscle wasting.

Tamoxifen (Nolvadex)

Low platelet count, usually mild and transient, leukopenia, anemia. Rash, redness. Nausea, vomiting, anorexia (may lead to weight loss), diarrhea or constipation. Vaginal bleeding or discharge, menstrual changes (amenorrhea, menstrual irregularities), itchiness of the vulva. Increased liver enzymes, backing up of bile. Depression, dizziness, light-headedness, headache, confusion, lassitude, fainting. Hot flashes, clots in veins, pulmonary embolism, fluid retention and edema. Retinopathy, corneal opacity. Hypercalcemia. Other: Tumor "flare" may occur in the first month of therapy, manifested as an increase in tumor-related symptoms, such as bone pain, increase in tumor size, erythema. Effects in pregnancy; classified as Category D.

Taxol

Diminished number of white blood cells, dose-limiting. Hypersensitivity manifested as low blood pressure, shortness of breath with bronchospasm, hives, abdominal and extremity pain, allergic swelling, sweating. Half of the reported reactions occurred within two to three minutes of initiation of treatment; they usually occurred with the first dose. The incidence is greater with shorter infusions. Inflammation of mucous membranes, dose-related and cumulative; nausea, vomiting, diarrhea, infrequent and mild; taste changes. Nerve damage in extremities, more frequent with longer infusions with doses over $170mg/m^2$, and in patients with a history of substantial alcohol use, diabetes, or diabetic neuropathy; transient muscle aches and joint pain with higher doses; rarely, transient paralytic ileus, generalized weakness, seizures. Slow heart rate, usually transient and asymptomatic; ventricular tachycardia, usually asymptomatic but potentially serious; atypical chest pain. Hair loss, universal, complete, and often sudden, between days 14 and 21; often affects all body hair. Other: fatigue, headaches, minor elevations in renal and hepatic function tests, elevation of serum triglycerides.

Testolactone, Testosterone, Trilostane (Thiotepa (TESPA, TSPA, N, N', N"-Triethylene-Thiophosphoramide)

Systemic effects may occur following intravesicular administration. Low white blood cell count, low platelet count, anemia. Hair loss (rare with conventional doses), hives, rash, itching, bronzing, redness and/or peeling of skin in patients receiving 900 mg/m^2 prior to bone marrow transplantation. Nausea and vomiting (preventable), anorexia, inflammation of the tongue (often severe with bone marrow transplantation doses), diarrhea. Elevated liver enzymes (usually mild and transient). Urinary (in patients receiving intravesicular thiotepa); abdominal pain, blood in the urine, hemorrhagic cystitis (rare); painful urination, frequency, urgency, ureteral obstruction and impairment of renal function (one case). Headache, dizziness; weakness of lower extremities, tingling sensations (with injection given into the cerebrospinal fluid); cognitive impairment (e.g., stupor, coma) is the dose-limiting toxicity of high-dose thiotepa (first observed at 1125 mg/m^2 and increasing in severity at higher doses). Shortness of breath (in patients receiving succinylcholine). Other: second malignancy (i.e., leukemia); pain at site of injection; impaired fertility (azospermia, amenorrhea, etc.).

Vinblastine (Velban, VLB, Velsar, Alkaban AQ)

Low white blood cell count, low platelet count, anemia. Hair loss; skin and soft tissue damage if fluid goes onto skin (the manufacturer recommends subcutaneous injection of hyaluronidase and application of heat to help disperse the drug); rash, photosensitivity. Nausea, vomiting (preventable); constipation (see neurological side effects); abdominal pain (cramps), anorexia, diarrhea, inflammation of mucous membranes, gastrointestinal hemorrhage. Nerve damage in extremities (loss of deep tendon reflexes, tingling sensations, paralysis); constipation, paralytic ileus, urinary retention, blood pressure changes due to position changes; vocal cord paralysis; muscle aches; Raynaud's phenomenon; headache, seizures, depression, dizziness, malaise; may be enhanced by concomitant use of interferon. Acute shortness of breath, more common when administered with mitomycin; pulmonary edema.

Other: severe pain in the jaw, pharynx, bones, back, or limbs following injection; fever; cardiotoxicity; enhanced interferon toxicity.

Vincristine (Oncovin, Vincasar, VCR, Leucocristine, LCR)

Low white blood cell count (mild and rare), low platelet count (rare), anemia. Hair loss; skin and soft tissue damage of tissues when solution goes into tissues (the manufacturer recommends subcutaneous injection of hyaluronidase and application of heat to help disperse the drug); rash. Nausea, vomiting (rare); constipation (see neurological side effects); abdominal pain (cramps); anorexia; diarrhea. Fatal ascending paralysis follows administration into the cerebrospinal fluid. Elevated liver enzymes (mild and transient). Nerve damage in extremities (loss of deep tendon reflexes, tingling sensations, paralysis); constipation, paralytic ileus, urinary retention, blood pressure changes due to position changes; unsteady gait; muscle aches; cortical blindness; headache; seizures. Acute shortness of breath, more common when administered with mitomycin. Ocular: double vision; ptosis; photophobia; cortical blindness; optic atrophy. Other: Severe pain in the jaw, pharynx, bones, back, and limbs following injection; fever pancreatitis (rare).

Glossary

adjuvant systemic therapy: anticancer drugs that are used in combination with surgery and/or radiation to prevent or delay cancer from spreading.

anesthesia: a procedure in which a patient receives medications that block out pain. General anesthesia also causes loss of consciousness.

anesthesiologist: a medical doctor specially trained to administer anesthesia.

aspiration: a procedure in which a hollow needle withdraws fluid from a breast mass into a syringe or vacuum tube.

autologous bone marrow transplant: removal of a person's bone marrow to allow for toxic chemotherapy; the same marrow (rather than a donor's) is replaced after the chemotherapy.

benign: without cancer. A benign or nonmalignant tumor is one that does not invade and destroy neighboring normal tissue, or spread to other parts of the body.

bone marrow: soft cell tissue in center of bones, where red and white blood cells are manufactured.

biopsy: removal of tissue to examine for cancer cells.

breast reduction: surgery to diminish the size of a breast.

cancer: a general term for diseases characterized by uncontrolled, abnormal growth of cells that can invade and destroy healthy tissues. Also called malignant neoplasm or malignancy.

care partner: a person who takes an active, supportive role throughout your treatment.

CAT scan: computerized axial tomography. Special computerized X-ray examination that allows for precise visualization of tumors. Rarely used to detect breast tumors.

chemotherapy: treatment with toxic chemicals capable of destroying cancer cells.

clinical trials: controlled studies to evaluate new treatments.

diagnosis: process of determining the nature of a disease. It is a necessary preliminary to treatment.

estrogen: a female sex hormone produced by the ovaries, adrenal glands, placenta, and fatty tissues.

expander: an empty sack that is placed behind the chest muscle and filled with saline over a period of months to stretch the skin before a breast implant is put in place.

flap procedure: reconstructive surgery that re-creates the normal shape of the breast using the patient's own body tissue.

frozen section: part of the biopsy tissue frozen immediately. A thin slice is then mounted on microscope slides and examined by a pathologist.

guided imagery: process of being helped to imagine a picture of an event, place or action. Also called visualization.

hormone therapy: treating cancer by removing or adding hormones.

implants: a breast replacement inserted surgically under the skin.

intraductal carcinoma in situ (DCIS): located in the milk ducts of the breast, this condition is believed to have a 30–40 percent lifetime chance of developing into infiltrating breast cancer.

intravenous (IV) infusion: slowly dripping fluids into a vein through a tube.

lesion: groups of cells or a mass; could apply to a lump, abscess, etc.

living will: a written form that describes how a person wants to be cared for and that names a surrogate decision maker, if s/he is unable to voice his or her wishes.

lobular carcinoma in situ (LCIS): considered precancer, this "marker" is located in the deeper areas where milk production starts. It is believed to carry a small risk—20 percent over a lifetime—of developing into infiltrating cancer.

lump: any kind of mass in the breast or elsewhere in the body.

lumpectomy: the surgical removal of a breast lump and a small area of surrounding tissue. This is also called partial mastectomy, quadranectomy, or wide excision.

lymphedema: a swelling that results from the removal of lymph nodes and the inability of the lymph system to drain fluid from the tissues.

lymph nodes: small glands containing white blood cells that remove wastes from body tissues and that help the body fight infection. They are examined by a pathologist after surgical removal to help determine the extent of disease.

malignant: cancerous.

mammogram: a low-dose X-ray photograph of the breast that can often detect tumors too small to be felt.

mastectomy: the surgical removal of the breast.

mastectomy (modified radical): the most common mastectomy procedure, this involves removal of the breast and the lymph nodes in the armpit.

mastectomy (partial, wide excision, or quadrantectomy): see **lumpectomy.**

mastectomy (radical or Halstead): rarely done, this involves the removal of the breast, muscles of the chest wall, and enough skin to require a skin graft.

mastectomy (simple): removal of breast tissue.

mediport: a temporary device that is surgically implanted in the chest or arm to accept an IV during chemotherapy.

megace: hormonal medication used in the treatment of advanced breast cancer.

metastasis: the spread of cancer cells from one location to another, usually through the bloodstream or lymph channels. Cells in the new cancer are like those in the original site.

oncologist: a physician who specializes in the treatment of cancer.

oncology: study, science, or treatment of cancer.

pathologist: a physician who specializes in the diagnosis of disease through the microscopic study of cells and tissue.

pathology: that part of medicine that deals with the results of disease and the changes that accompany it, particularly as seen in cells, organs, and tissues.

pathology report: the pathologist's written record of the analysis of the tissue.

phantom sensation: the feeling that a body part is present, even after it has been removed.

plastic surgeon: a medical doctor specially trained to do cosmetic and reconstructive surgery.

prognosis: doctor's forecast of the probable course of a disease.

prosthesis: any artificial substitute for a missing body part; here, an artificial breast form that can be worn under clothing after a mastectomy.

protocol: the course of treatment being used.

radiation oncologist: a doctor who specializes in using radiation to treat cancer.

radiation therapy: high-energy, localized X-rays used to destroy cancer cells.

radiologist: a medical doctor who specializes in the interpretation of X-rays for diagnosis and treatment.

Reach to Recovery: a national program sponsored by the American Cancer Society in which women who have had breast surgery visit and counsel women after surgery, providing practical information, a temporary prosthesis, and some exercise suggestions.

reconstructive surgery: plastic surgery that re-creates the normal shape of the breasts.

recurrence: reappearance of cancer at the same site (local), near the initial site (regional), or in other areas of the body (metastatic).

relaxation: the reduction of tension.

saline: a sterile saltwater solution.

sedative: medication that has a tranquilizing effect.

silicone: a synthetic material used to encase and fill some breast implants.

sonogram: the image created by ultrasound examination.

Tamoxifen (Nolvadex®): an estrogen blocker used to treat breast cancer.

teaching hospital: a hospital affiliated with a medical school.

toxic: poisonous.

TRAM-flap procedure: reconstructive surgery that re-creates the normal shape of the breasts using abdominal tissue.

tumor: an abnormal growth of cells or tissue. Swelling or enlargement due to abnormal overgrowth of tissue. Tumors can either be benign or malignant.

two-step procedure: biopsy and treatment performed at two different times.

ultrasound: a painless test using high-frequency sound waves to determine whether a lump is liquid or solid.

Zoladex: medication that stops estrogen production.

About the Authors

Joan Swirsky, R.N., M.S., C.S., ACCE, is a clinical nurse specialist in psychiatric–mental health nursing, and an ASPO-certified childbirth educator. She received the Master's Faculty Leadership Award from Adelphi University and is a member of Sigma Theta Tau Nursing Honor Society.

The recipient of seven Long Island Press Awards, Ms. Swirsky writes for the *New York Times* (Long Island Section), the *Women's Record* (a Long Island monthly magazine), and a variety of other publications. For her extensive writing and political activism on the issue of breast cancer on Long Island, she has received citations from Nassau County and the Town of North Hempstead, and was the recipient of the first annual Benita Feurey Award from the Adelphi University School of Social Work Oncology Support Program and the Long Island Breast Cancer Coalition. She was appointed by Governor Cuomo to membership on the New York State Breast Cancer Advisory Board.

Ms. Swirsky is the author and editor of *Nurse Abuse: Impact and Resolution* and the editor-in-chief of a national nursing magazine, *Revolution: The Journal of Nurse Empowerment,* which made its debut in January 1992. She and her husband, Steve, who is the president of a manufacturer's representative agency, have three grown children.

Barbara Balaban, A.C.S.W., BCD, is a social worker and life-long activist. She is director of the Breast Cancer Hotline and Support Program at Adelphi University's School of Social Work in Garden City, New York, where she also teaches part-time. The Breast Cancer Support Program runs New York's Statewide Breast Cancer Hotline, provides breast cancer support groups, engages in patient, community, and professional education programs, and coordinates New York State breast cancer grass roots activities for the National Breast Cancer Coalition.

Ms. Balaban received the master's degree in social welfare from the State University of New York at Stony Brook and is a graduate of both the Training Program of the Ackerman Institute for Family Therapy and the Behavior Therapy Training Program at Cornell Medical School.

A founder of the breast cancer advocacy movement on Long Island, she was a member of the Center for Disease Control's panel on "Breast Cancer on Long Island" to investigate the high incidence of breast cancer on Long Island. She also chairs the Long Island Breast Cancer Coalition, serves on the Nassau County Breast Cancer Steering Committee, and is a board member of the National Breast Cancer Coalition, serving as national secretary for that group.

Ms. Balaban was named Woman of Record in 1992 by the *Women's Record* and Social Worker of the Year in 1993 by the Suffolk County Division of the National Association of Social Workers.

She and her husband, Al, have three grown children, two in-laws, and five grandchildren.